STRONGER

STRONGER

Jeff Bauman

with Bret Witter

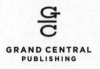

GRAND CENTRAL
PUBLISHING

NEW YORK   BOSTON

Grand Central Publishing
Hachette Book Group
1290 Avenue of the Americas
New York, NY 10104

GrandCentralPublishing.com

Printed in the United States of America

RRD-C

Originally published in hardcover by Grand Central Publishing.

First trade edition: December 2014

10 9 8 7 6 5 4 3 2 1

Grand Central Publishing is a division of Hachette Book Group, Inc. The Grand Central Publishing name and logo is a trademark of Hachette Book Group, Inc.

The Hachette Speakers Bureau provides a wide range of authors for speaking events. To find out more, go to www.hachettespeakersbureau.com or call (866) 376-6591.

The publisher is not responsible for websites (or their content) that are not owned by the publisher.

LCCN 2013050788

ISBN 978-1-4555-8436-9 (pbk.)

To Mom and Dad

STRONGER

THE BOMB

·◆·

April 15, 2013

I know exactly when my life changed: when I looked into the face of Tamerlan Tsarnaev. It was 2:48 p.m. on April 15, 2013—one minute before the most high-profile terrorist event on United States soil since September 11—and he was standing right beside me.

We were half a block from the finish line of the Boston Marathon, two in a crowd of half a million. The marathon was the signature event of Patriot's Day, Boston's special holiday, which celebrates Paul Revere's ride and the local militiamen who fought the first battle of the American Revolution on April 19, 1775. Patriot's Day was also the unofficial start of spring, in a city known for brutal winters, so half the city had taken the day off, and everyone wanted to be outside. By tradition, a Red Sox home game had started at 11:00 a.m., coinciding with the last starting group of the marathon. By 2:30, baseball fans were pouring out of Yawkey Way onto Boylston Street, swelling the marathon crowd.

I had arrived half an hour earlier, with my friends Remy and Michele, to cheer for my girlfriend, Erin Hurley. Even then, the sidewalks were clogged ten deep, and the restaurants and bars were filled with people in Red Sox gear and Boston shirts. The best runners, who qualified for the first start time, had finished hours before, but the runners kept coming, and the crowd kept growing. Most of these people, including Erin, were running for charity. They were the average runners, the ones who needed and deserved our support. Everywhere I looked, people were cheering and clapping, yelling for them to keep going, the finish line was close, they were almost there.

And then I noticed Tsarnaev.

I don't know how he got beside me. I just remember looking over my right shoulder and seeing him. He was standing close, maybe a foot away, and there was something off about him. He was wearing sunglasses and a white baseball cap pulled low over his face, and he had on a hooded jacket that seemed too heavy, even on a cool day. The thing that really struck me, though, was his demeanor. Everyone was cheering and watching the race. Everyone was enjoying themselves. Except this guy. He was alone, and he wasn't having a good time.

He was all business.

He turned toward me. I couldn't see his eyes, because of his sunglasses, but I know he was staring at me. I know now he was planning to kill me—in less than a minute, he thought I'd be dead—but his face revealed no emotion. No doubt. No remorse. The guy was a rock.

We stared at each other for eight, maybe ten seconds, then my friend Michele said something, and I turned to talk to her. Our friend Remy had moved toward the finish line to try to get a better view. I was about to suggest to Michele that we join her. That was how much this guy bothered me.

But I didn't. And when I looked back, he was gone.

Thank God, I thought. . . .

Until I noticed his backpack. It was sitting on the ground, near my feet. I felt a jolt of fear, and that old airport warning started running through my head: Don't leave bags unattended. Report suspicious packages. I looked around, hoping to find the guy—

And then I heard it. The explosion. Not like a bomb in a movie, not a big bang, but three pops, one after the other.

It doesn't get hazy after that. It gets very clear. The hospital psychiatrist later told me that my brain "lit up," that at the moment the bomb went off my brain became hyperalert, so that even though my memories are fragmented into hundreds of pieces, all the pieces are clear.

I remember opening my eyes and seeing smoke, then realizing I was on the ground looking up at the sky.

I remember a woman stepping over me, covered in blood. Then others, scattering in all directions.

There was blood on the ground. Chunks of flesh. And heat. There was a terrible amount of heat. It smelled like a cookout in hell.

There was an accident, I thought. Something went wrong.

I sat up. Michele was lying on her back a few feet away, a race barrier collapsed on top of her. I could see her bone through a hole in her lower leg.

That's not good, I thought.

We made eye contact. She reached toward me, and I started to reach toward her. Then she looked at my legs, and she stopped, and her eyes got wide.

I looked down. There was nothing below my knees. I was sitting in a chunky pool of blood—my blood—and my lower legs were gone.

I looked around. Blood was everywhere. Body parts were everywhere, and not just mine.

This wasn't an accident, I thought. He did this to us. That fucker did this to us.

Then I heard the second explosion, somewhere in the distance. It had only been twelve seconds since the first bomb went off.

This is a war, I thought. They're going to chase him. There's going to be shooting. They won't be able to get to me.

I lay down. I'm going to die, I thought, and I realized I was okay with that. I had lived a short life, only twenty-seven years, but a good life. I was okay with letting go.

Then an emergency room surgeon named Allen Panter, who had been watching the race from across the street, appeared above me. He slammed tourniquets around the ragged ends where my legs had been blown off, yelling as he worked.

"Get shirts!" he was screaming over his shoulder. "Get jackets! Shoelaces! Anything! People are bleeding out here!"

"Get away from me," I said.

"Stay calm."

I had been calm. I had been completely calm. But this guy was freaking me out. "Go help someone else!" I yelled, pushing him away. "Go help my friend!"

He dipped his hand in my blood and drew a red "C" on my forehead. I remember that so clearly. I think it meant "critical."

Then he was gone, yelling orders as he went. My ears were ringing, but I could still hear the screaming.

I saw a woman lying motionless, her eyes open.

I saw a man in a yellow cowboy hat lift the barrier off Michele, then turn toward me, and the next thing I knew he was grabbing my shirt and twisting it around his fist. He lifted me off the ground with one hand, spun around, and threw me into a wheelchair that had been intended for runners too tired to walk after finishing the race.

When I hit the chair, it was an electric shock. It was like that scene in *Pulp Fiction*, when John Travolta plunged the adrenaline into Uma Thurman's heart. My body came alive, and I thought, No way, Jeff. No way that fucker is taking you down.

"I'm going to make it," I said.

"Yeah, buddy," the man in the cowboy hat said, running beside me. "That's right. You're going to make it."

We passed through a medical tent. People were yelling for us to stop.

"No!" the man yelled without slowing down. "We're going to the hospital."

The tourniquet on my right leg pulled loose. It got stuck in the wheel and tore off, and suddenly there was a second man there, and the two of them were holding my right leg and squeezing to stop the bleeding. I reached down and grabbed my left leg, trying to do the same. A photographer appeared out of the chaos, kneeling in the road as we rushed past, snapping pictures.

I thought, What is he doing here?

We crossed the finish line of the Boston Marathon. I saw the banner as I was lifted out of the wheelchair and into an ambulance.

"Who are you?" a woman said. "What is your name?"

"I'm Bauman," I said as they strapped me down. "Jeff Bauman."

"Are you Bowman?" the woman yelled at the man in the cowboy hat.

"What?"

"Are you Bowman?"

"No," he said, misunderstanding my name. "I'm not his brother."

And then we were gone, racing up Boylston Street toward Boston Medical Center while an EMT worked on my legs.

"I know what happened," I said.

The EMT hesitated, looking at my face for the first time. "He's awake," he yelled to someone in the front seat. "This guy's still awake."

"It was a bomb," I said.

"Are you sure?"

"Yes. It was a bomb."

"How do you know?"

"I saw the guy. I know who did it."

I slipped out of consciousness for a second, maybe two, then jerked awake. Don't do that, Jeff, I told myself. Stay alert.

I remember everything. The equipment hanging above me in the ambulance. The orderlies waiting when we arrived. I remember being rushed down a hallway, a policeman in uniform running beside me.

I know who did it, I tried to tell him. *I know. I know.* And I wanted someone else to know, just in case. But I couldn't get him to stop. I couldn't get anyone to listen.

"Stay calm," people kept saying. "Lie down and stay calm."

And then I was on the operating table, with ten or twelve people standing above me. That was when I started to panic. I've seen a lot of hospitals on television and in movies. I don't like hospitals.

"Put me under," I yelled. "I'm awake. Put me under."

A face came toward me, in front of the others. He was a young guy. He looked like Major Winters from *Band of Brothers*. "Don't worry," he said. "We'll take care of you."

And they did. Everyone that day took care of me. They saved my life. They are the heroes, because they gave me this opportunity. They gave me the chance to prove that I—that we—are better than cowards with bombs. That we're not broken. And we're not afraid.

We're stronger.

BEFORE

1.

Chelmsford, Massachusetts, is twenty-four miles from downtown Boston, near the manufacturing city of Lowell. It's known around Boston as a commuter suburb, but some people come here for the history, I guess. Chelmsford was a textile center in the 1820s, and a lot of the mills on the north side of town have been converted into shopping malls and condos. The downtown common, Chelmsford Center, is surrounded by old clapboard buildings: the Central Baptist Church, the Chelmsford Center for the Arts, and the First Parish Unitarian Universalist Church, built in 1660, current structure 1842. All Are Welcome, according to the small sign out front. Nearby are a one-room schoolhouse (1802) and the Middlesex Canal House (1832). The Forefathers Burial Ground (1655) is wedged between the common and a strip mall featuring a Bertucci's and my favorite local coffee joint, the Java Room.

Of course, I've only been in town since 1989, when I was two years old, so my personal history with the place doesn't involve old mills or clapboard churches, or the Merrimack River that brought the mills in the first place. My landmarks are more like Zesty's Pizza, the best place in town for a slice. Sully's, near the high school, which has the best ice cream. The Brickhouse, a bar with good subs across from the Unitarian Church, where all are also welcome, as long as they're Red Sox fans. And, of course, Hong Kong Chinese American Food, whose huge neon sign towers above the parking lot of the Radisson. The Hong Kong is my aunt Jenn's favorite place. She's been drinking there since she was sixteen, so the place must be ancient, probably from the 1970s. It has egg rolls, but it's known for its dance floor and mai tais. I think every suburb of Boston has a place like the Hong Kong.

I admit, I used to go to the Hong Kong with Aunt Jenn and Big D (my cousin Derek). It's a Chelmsford institution. Then one night, about a year before the bombing, Vinnie the bartender, who is Chinese despite the name and seems to have worked at the Hong Kong every night since 1982, pointed at one of my high school friends, who was drunk and doing the worst dance I'd ever seen. "He don't come back," Vinnie said.

I thought, Maybe it's time I moved on from this place, too.

It wasn't that I didn't enjoy my life. Far from it. I loved my life, even if it wasn't always easy. I was born in South Jersey, near Philly, but my parents divorced when I was two. It wasn't a pleasant divorce. Mom, angry and heartbroken, moved home to be near her family, but she struggled, especially financially, like a lot of single moms. She worked double shifts as a waitress. She took on odd jobs. She worried: about me, about all the time she had to spend away from me, about our future. We lived in four or five different apartments when I was growing up; every month, Mom worried about the rent.

She liked to drink. Some in the family want to make more of it than that, like maybe she needed drinking to take the edge off, but that was the way I always saw it: Mom liked to drink. Never during the day, but every night. Sometimes when she was out with her younger sister, Aunt Jenn, or sometimes when she was with friends. Other times it was at home alone. What can I say about it? I'm her kid. I never knew anything else.

My dad, Big Jeff, stayed in my life. He fought for visitation rights. When I was nine, he moved to Concord, New Hampshire, an hour and a half from Chelmsford, to be closer to me. He had married his high school sweetheart after the divorce, and he had a new family: two step-daughters and two more sons. I spent weeks with him in the summer, and I tried to be there whenever my half brothers, Chris and Alan, had a hockey game. I will never forget my dad's wife, Big Csilla, taking me strawberry picking. She was always kind.

But it was Mom, and her brother and sisters, who raised me. It was Christmas at their father's house, with the Cavit wine flowing, that I remember most. After Grandpa died, Mom's brother, Uncle Bob, took Mom and me in for a year and a half, and her sisters, Aunt Karen and Aunt Jenn, let me live with each of them for a while when I was in high school. Aunt Jenn was sixteen years older than me, but she acted like my big sister. She was always taking me and Big D out shopping or to the movies and later, when we were older, to the dreaded Hong Kong.

We stuck together. I guess that's what I'm saying. There was always a family barbecue or birthday party to attend, and if we got rowdy, or ended up arguing, there was always a Red Sox, Patriots, Celtics, or Bruins game on television, and the perfect chance to sit around and laugh together about whatever we had done.

Uncle Bob even had Red Sox season tickets for a while, back before everyone became a fan. He gave me and Big D his tickets to Game 4 of the 2004 American League Championship series. That was the night the Red Sox, down three games to none to the New York Yankees—no team had ever come back from three games to none in a baseball play-off series—turned around eighty-six years of futility. We were in the upper deck, but with the Red Sox losing in the late innings, everyone in front of us started leaving, so we moved closer. We kept moving closer, then closer, until we were right next to the field. We were practically in the on-deck circle by the ninth inning, when Dave Roberts stole second base.

I was seventeen years old; Big D was sixteen. I didn't have much, materially speaking, but what more do you need when the Red Sox come back in the last inning off the best closer in the history of baseball, Mariano Rivera, and you're there? You are there. Only a few feet away.

I went to Middlesex Community College the next year, but I didn't make it through. So Uncle Bob took me in at his paving company. Uncle Bob was completely irreverent, and often inappropriate, but he was smart as hell. He'd built his paving business from scratch. Big D and I were known as the family cutups, always in the corner at family functions, cracking jokes. Having a good time. But we learned that from Uncle Bob, who couldn't go five minutes without a wisecrack, usually at Aunt Jenn's expense.

"Give Jeff a taco," Aunt Jenn would say, trying to be serious, "and he's happy. That kid doesn't need much."

"As long as he doesn't get the taco from you." Uncle Bob would laugh.

"Yeah, you make the Hong Kong's food look good, Aunt Jenn."

"And I wouldn't eat there if you paid me," Big D would add.

"I wouldn't even step foot in there before ten o'clock."

"And nothing good ever happens at the Hong Kong after ten o'clock."

"That's Aunt Jenn time."

I loved Uncle Bob—he was like a father to me—but I didn't want to work in the family business. I wanted my own career. So after a few years, I went back to college at the University of Massachusetts Lowell. I took mostly math and science courses, with the goal of becoming an engineer. Engineers can make $70,000 a year.

That didn't work out, either. I had student loans to cover most of my costs, but somehow I ended up owing $900, and I couldn't register for the next semester.

I didn't have $900. At that point in my life, I don't think I'd ever had $900, and I doubt Mom had, either. I could have asked Uncle Bob for it, and he'd probably have given it to me. But Mom had taught me to be self-reliant. You can take something from people who love you, but you never ask for it. Besides, I'd started working part-time in the deli at Costco. I figured I'd take another semester off, work at Costco, and see if I could save $900.

Three years later, I was still working at the Costco deli counter. It wasn't my career, I knew that, but I enjoyed it. The work was easy, mostly prep and stocking food cases, and I loved my coworkers, from my supervisor, Maya, right up to "Heavy Kevy," who managed the store. Kevin Horst was actually six foot four and maybe 180 pounds. He was in great shape, and he was immaculate. I didn't know Kevin well, because he managed almost two hundred employees, but I knew you couldn't put a piece of lettuce out of place on a salad without Kevin noticing.

I never saved that $900 for college. Costco kept me below forty hours a week, a standard practice in retail, so I was making less than $16,000 a year. I was sharing an apartment with Sully, my best friend since third grade, and his girlfriend, Jill, and I was still barely breaking even. Then Sully and Jill broke up, and we couldn't afford the apartment, so I moved back in with Mom.

It was a typical move in my life. Easy. Because of my childhood, I'd never gotten too attached to a space, and I never accumulated much stuff. Even at twenty-six, I didn't own a computer. I didn't have a possession to my name except a cell phone, a guitar my grandmother had given me a $100 check to buy on my eighteenth birthday, and a twelve-year-old Volkswagen Passat. I drove the Passat an hour to Concord, New Hampshire, every other week to visit my dad. He fixed transmissions at AAMCO, and they let him use the shop after hours. That was the only way we kept my beat-up car on the road.

It was a great life. A great, great life. I was happy. I had my own car, my own room, and enough money for an occasional trip to Boston. I had a bunch of friends from high school, so I was out every evening before Mom got home from the dinner shift. And because I didn't have anything, nobody asked me for anything. They let me be who I was: a quiet kid. Happy-go-lucky. Always trying to make sure everyone had a good time. I was young. I didn't know where I was going, but I knew I was in no hurry to get there.

Then I met Erin.

It was May 2012, eleven months before the bombing, and a few weeks after I'd sworn off the Hong Kong for the eleven hundredth time. Some friends and I had gone into Boston to see ALO, one of my favorite bands. Afterward, we went to a party at someone's house, and Erin was there. She was easy to be around. Interesting. Beautiful. We hit it off right away. She later told me what she liked most about me was that I was so nice.

Ouch, E. That kind of stings.

Unfortunately, Erin lived an hour away in Brighton, an in-town Boston neighborhood that's the kind of place you live after you graduate from college and before you have kids. It was a commute, but I knew after our first date—Flatbread Pizza in Somerville, followed by *Prometheus*, in hindsight not the most romantic movie choice—that she was worth it.

Erin wasn't like my friends in Chelmsford. She had been born in Alabama and raised in Amesbury, Massachusetts, in a house with solar panels and a wood stove. She graduated from Lesley University, a mostly girls' college in Cambridge, where she ran cross-country and met Michele, my future fellow bombing victim. Erin had a career. She was a program coordinator in the anesthesiology department at Brigham and Women's Hospital downtown, and she was planning to go back to school for a master's degree in health administration. Her boss wanted to promote her. Erin just needed the degree first.

Unfortunately, our schedules were a mess. She worked a typical eight-to-six. I usually worked the closing shift at Costco, so I didn't get off until after 8:30. That meant I couldn't get to Brighton until ten, about the time Erin was getting ready for bed, since she had to get up at 6:30 for work. And I worked weekends, too, so we often went weeks without a good chunk of time together.

But we made it work. I spent nights in Boston with Erin and her roommates: Remy, her best childhood friend, and Michele, her best college friend. We discovered favorite bars and coffee joints. We went to Washington, D.C. We went on an overnight rafting trip to Maine, something I had been wanting to do for years. When the junk shop at the end of Erin's block turned into a takeout chicken wing counter, it felt like destiny.

"She's so nice," Mom said, every time Erin stayed over in Chelmsford.

Ha-ha, E, that word got you, too!

But it's true. Erin is nice. She's not a party girl, but get a few beers in her and she'll break out the dance moves. I guess it would make you uncomfortable if I said sexy, right, E? But it's true. Erin puts the sexy in nice. But she preferred a nice quiet home-cooked meal, and a nice quiet life.

In August, with the relationship heating up, I invited Erin to my nephew Cole's seventh birthday party. This was a big deal, because Cole's birthday was the event of the summer for my extended family. Aunt Jenn was older when she had Cole—she was Uncle Dale's third wife—so she spoiled him. Even she admits it. For his birthday, she gets the jumpy house, and the catered barbecue, and invites everyone. There are usually eighty people at Cole's birthday party, most of them relatives.

Fortunately, I was working at Costco that Saturday, so Erin and I had an excuse to show up late, after most of the guests had left. This was, after all, the first girlfriend I'd introduced to the whole family. I hadn't had to before. Most of my past girlfriends had been around my family forever.

"Great girl," Uncle Bob said, in one of his rare serious moments. "Good head on her shoulders."

By which he meant: She had a plan. She was going places.

And she was. Erin had worked her way through college. She was successful, and she was going to be more successful in the future. She wanted that for me, too. She never judged me because I didn't make much money and lived with my mom. She didn't care about that.

But she believed in me. She wanted me to finish college. She thought I had a future as an engineer.

"Maybe next year," I told her. "When you go to grad school, I'll go back to college. We can study together."

I meant it, except maybe for the studying. I'd been telling Mom I'd go back to college for years, but Erin made me see it as something I shouldn't just say. If we were going to have a life together, it was something I should do.

But then, sometime that winter, we started to drift apart. Maybe I got cold feet, I don't know, but I started to skip trips down to Boston to visit her. After six months, I told myself I was tired of the drive. I was cooking chicken and ribs all day at Costco. I was helping customers. I wanted to go home after my shift and relax. Play some guitar in my room. Watch a Bruins hockey game with Sully and Big D.

Erin was frustrated that I kept breaking dates. "I changed my plans to be with you," she'd say.

"I'm sorry," I'd say. "I'm tired."

We talked about moving in together, so we wouldn't have to commute to see each other, but that would have meant quitting my job, so nothing came of it.

"You aren't really committed," Erin would say. It wasn't a complaint. It was a statement of fact.

"You need to do what you say you're going to do," she would tell me. "If you make a promise, you need to be there."

That was big for Erin. She was a planner. She loved a routine. She had always been a runner, but that winter she was training for the Boston Marathon. Brigham and Women's needed to upgrade their neonatal intensive care unit, so a group from the hospital was running to raise money.

"It feels good to be helping," she said. But it also meant less time together.

That Christmas, I bought Erin a nice camera at Costco. A few weeks later, I bought myself a guitar. It was a Yamaha Acoustic Electric, on sale at Guitar Center for $200, and I couldn't resist. That's a bargain.

I've always loved playing guitar. Nothing too serious. I just find it relaxing. I'd jam with my half brother Chris on my dad's back porch in Concord, New Hampshire, or sit in my room and work on songs. I knew some guys who played at clubs in downtown Lowell, the center of the local music scene, so I started heading down there to the open mic nights with my friend Blair. I wouldn't play. I was more of a listener. Blair would yell at the bands. We'd drink a few beers, and maybe a few too many. I've never been into any other type of drug or alcohol. I like beer.

"It's fine to go out and have a good time with your friends," Erin said. "I want you to do that. But not all the time."

She was right. When I first started skipping visits to Boston, it was because I was tired. Now I was skipping Erin to drink and listen to music with Blair.

"I can't do it," I told him next time he called. "I got plans."

But . . . I don't know. It wasn't enough. Erin and I were having a great time together, but it wasn't enough. I kept screwing up. I remember one day in February, the dead of winter, heading up to my dad's house in New Hampshire and walking in the door with the usual twelve-pack under my arm.

"What's happenin', Big Csilla?" (It's pronounced "Big Chilla." My stepsister, Little Csilla, has the same name.)

She could tell right away something was wrong. "Where's Erin?"

"Ah, we broke up."

"What happened?"

"I broke one too many promises."

I don't like talking about personal stuff, so that's what I said, over and over again, since everyone in my family had to ask. We broke up. I had called Erin two days after. I told her I loved her. She said it wasn't enough.

I didn't see her again until March 29. That was the day of her marathon fund-raiser at Sissy K's, a bar in Brighton. We had talked about the fund-raiser a lot, and she had worked on it for months, so I knew it was important to her. That was why I came—to support her. I even brought Big D and Aunt Jenn. There was dancing and a DJ. How could I not bring Aunt Jenn?

I didn't realize how much I wanted to be there until I saw Erin. She wasn't expecting me, but she smiled as soon as I walked in. I could tell she wanted me there, and that was when I realized the only place I wanted to be was with her.

I don't remember our conversation. When she asked what I was doing there, I think I just said, "I told you I'd come."

We left the party together, and that was that.

Two weeks later, Erin woke me up at 5:00 a.m. It was Monday, April 15, 2013, Patriot's Day, and the day of the Boston Marathon. As planned, I drove Erin to Hopkinton, where the race buses would take the runners to the starting line. It was hours before the first wave of runners, those in wheelchairs, started at 9:40. Erin was in the third wave, starting at 10:40, but there were already twenty thousand runners milling about, ready to go.

"You better win," I told her as I kissed her good-bye. She laughed. Then I went back to her apartment and went to bed.

I saw her again around 1:30, near mile 18 in Newton. Remy, Michele, and I had told her to look for us there, near the start of Heartbreak Hill, the hardest climb on the course. I had a poster-board sign that said: "Run E(rin) Run!" Remy and Michele had oversized fans for Team Stork, the charity Erin was raising money for.

We pushed through the crowds lining both sides of the street until we could see the runners streaming past. The fire station down the block had a live band, and people were dancing and cheering. Two soldiers with rucksacks marched past, raising money for veterans. Another dude was running in a hamburger costume; I have no idea why. I had never been to the marathon before. I'd seen it on television, but I hadn't been in the crowd. Being there made me realize how special it was. The race was 137 years old, the oldest continuously held marathon in the world. It was huge, and it was ours. Our holiday. Our tradition. Our pride. It wasn't just a sporting event, I realized; it was a celebration. Winter was over, it was a beautiful day, and everyone was alive and dancing.

In fact, Remy, Michele, and I were having so much fun, we almost missed Erin. We noticed her right as she passed us, and we had to chase her, yelling her name. She circled back and gave us a group hug, smiling, even though she was exhausted.

"I'll see you at the finish line," I said, giving her a kiss.

Erin nodded. "I'll be there."

And then she was gone, up the slope toward Heartbreak Hill. It seemed so trivial at the time, like the most ordinary thing in the world. I guess that's usually how it is before bad luck, or random chance, changes your life.

FIRST DAYS

2.

The bomb went off at 2:49 on Monday afternoon. Within seconds, the man in the cowboy hat was leaping the barricade guarding the finish line and racing toward the carnage. The second bomb went off when he was halfway across the street, but he kept coming. They all kept coming to help us: police officers, race volunteers, bystanders.

Strangers were huddled over victims on the ground, assuring them that it would be all right, that help was on the way, that they weren't alone. People were stripping off sweaters and belts for tourniquets. Some held wounds closed with their hands. The Boston bomb squad ripped into backpacks and packages with knives, a so-called "slash-and-tag." They figured if there were two bombs, there probably was a third to kill the people trying to help. That was usually how terrorist attacks worked. A "slash-and-tag" on a third bomb would probably kill the bomb squad officer, but it would save other lives.

At first, it was reported as an electrical fire, or maybe a sewer explosion. Manhole covers sometimes blew off without warning. But it didn't take long for word of bombs to spread. Posts and tweets from the scene. Cell phone pictures of blood on the streets. Boston is a small city, about one-sixth the size of New York City. Within minutes, everyone was on social media, trying to find out if their friends were okay.

No one could reach me. Family and friends called and texted, but there was no answer. The bomb had either shattered my cell phone or sent it flying. I remember trying to find it when I was on the ground. I wanted to call Mom and tell her good-bye, don't worry, I'm not suffering, I'm just going now, I had a good life.

But the phone was gone. I couldn't reach anyone, and no one could reach me. Then they shut down the towers, and all the cell phones went dead.

The first pictures came out almost immediately thereafter. They were long shots of the scene: The concussion from the bomb blast shaking a camera that had been filming the race. The force of the blast knocking down a runner about to cross the finish line. The plume of smoke.

Then the first photo of a recognizable human face: my face. It was the now-famous photo of me in the wheelchair, with the man in the cowboy hat running beside me. Everyone calls it "iconic" now, but at the time it was horrifying. I had a cut above my eye, and one on my cheek. My face was pale and filthy from powder burns. My shirt was charred and bloodstained. And I had no legs.

Above the knees, I looked like any victim of a tragedy. It could have been a house fire, or a vicious brawl, that injured me. Below the knee, my legs were gone. Not shattered, but completely blown off. The only things remaining were a few pieces of ragged flesh and one long thin bone sticking down from my left knee.

Thanks to the man in the cowboy hat, I was the first victim to leave the scene of the bombing and the first to reach Boston Medical Center, less than two miles away. Within fifteen minutes, I was on the operating table, the emergency room surgeons slicing off the ripped ends of my legs and cauterizing my wounds. That saved my life.

And yet the photograph was faster. Even as the surgeons sawed into me, my face was popping up on websites. Someone recognized me and posted it to my Facebook page. Word started to spread among my friends. Before long, the photo was being shown on news reports.

My cousin Derek was paving roads with one of Uncle Bob's crews. He saw it on his break. "I couldn't breathe," Big D told me later. "I could not even breathe."

Aunt Jenn saw it at the zoo, where she had taken Cole to celebrate Patriot's Day. She immediately took him home. She has never let him look at the photo.

Sully clicked on my Facebook page and saw a cropped version, the one that shows me only from the waist up. Then he clicked on another site and saw my legs. He screamed, he told me, and fell to the floor.

My stepsister Erika saw it on television at the restaurant where she was waitressing. She called my dad at AAMCO. "Dad, Dad, did you see the picture? Jeffrey's on the news. He's hurt."

"Are you sure?" my dad shouted. He kept shouting until he found the photo online, and then he started to cry.

They even saw it at the Costco where I worked. They were watching bombing coverage in the break room, when my picture suddenly appeared. They couldn't reach me, so "Heavy Kevy" called the other phone number on file.

It was Mom. She was finishing her lunch shift and hadn't paid much attention to the bombing. She didn't even remember I had gone to the race. Typical Mom.

"No, I haven't heard from Jeff," she told Kevin. "Why?"

"He was at the marathon."

It dawned on her then. "Oh no, did he get hurt? Did he get hurt?"

"I think he might have."

"Is he alive?" she screamed. "Tell me, is he alive?"

"I don't—"

"What do you mean? What happened? Is my son alive?!"

"I don't know his condition. I'm sorry. But he is alive. I think you need to call the hospitals."

By then, Mom was hysterical. She put her friend on the phone, went to an empty table, and started crying.

Soon after, Aunt Cathleen, Uncle Bob's wife, called her. "I'm coming to get you," she said.

"Is Jeff all right? Please tell me Jeff is all right."

"I don't know," she said. "He's alive. There's a photo. I can't look at it. Bob said it's bad."

"That's not my son," Mom said, when she finally saw the photo an hour later. By then, she was back home. "That is not my son," she said. My face was so pale and scorched, it didn't even look like me.

"That's him, Patty," Aunt Cathleen said, putting a hand on her shoulder. "Look. That's his favorite shirt."

That afternoon was chaos. Complete chaos. I'm sure it was chaos all over the city, but especially in my family. Uncle Bob called doctors, trying to get a medical opinion based on the photograph. Mom's sisters called each other for information and support. They called every hospital in Boston, again and again, but without any luck—nobody could find me. Mom and Aunt Cathleen went to the local police station, desperate for news. Even the police couldn't help.

Finally, someone at Boston Medical Center said, "Wait. We have someone here with a similar name."

I had told them my name twenty times in the ambulance. They still wrote it down wrong when they admitted me.

So it was five hours until my family finally arrived at Boston Medical Center and learned what had happened to me. Five hours of trying not to stare at that photograph. Five hours of hearing about me on the news, knowing I was gravely injured, and not being able to find out anything more. In other words, five hours of fear.

A lot of people in the media were unsettled by the photo. They thought it violated my right to privacy, because I never consented to its use. They thought the uncropped version was too gruesome, even as a chronicle of a major event. After the initial rush, and often during it, most news sources used the cropped version, or they put a black bar over my lower left leg where the bone was exposed. Some, like the website for the *Atlantic*, showed the whole picture but pixilated my face so I wasn't recognizable.

But the graphic image was out there. It was the talk of Boston, and maybe beyond. For the rest of the day, whenever people huddled together to talk about the bombing, they talked about me: "Did you see the man in the wheelchair? The one without his legs?"

That was the shorthand people used when they wanted to share their horror. In those first hours, that was the image that brought the tragedy home.

The photograph doesn't bother me. I wish my family hadn't found out that way; I wish I was just another anonymous victim. The photo changed my life.

But that's the world we live in. A lot of people take pictures of a lot less interesting stuff. There are photos of me standing near the finish line before the bomb went off, and even photos of me on the ground. Charles Krupa, who took the iconic photo, worked for the Associated Press. I'm not upset with him. Why would I be mad at a journalist for doing his job? I'm mad that some kids set off a bomb. I'm mad that I lost my legs, and that a lot of people who have since become my friends lost their legs, too. I'm mad that three people were killed, including an eight-year-old boy.

But the photograph? It just showed what happened. A bomb exploded. It was packed with nails and ball bearings, which ripped through bodies, tore apart muscles, and shattered bones. It was built for maximum violence, and it worked. People were hurt in ways so horrible that seeing it makes you sick. I'm fine that the world was shocked, because bombing a crowd of innocent people is shocking.

But that's not what the photo is about. Not really. It doesn't show the bomb, and it doesn't show me being injured. It shows what happened afterward: Brave people rushed in. They saved our lives. Three people died at the scene. But nobody died at the hospital, or on the way to the hospital. Nobody died from bomb wounds over the next few weeks. There were 260 of us injured, and thanks to the bravery of others, we all have a chance to go on: to love and laugh and inspire, just like before.

That's why the picture doesn't bother me. Because it's not a picture of heartbreak, even though it's still too painful for me to see. It's a picture of hope, because the kid without his legs? The one burned and cut and deathly pale? He lived.

And he's going to be fine.

3.

The one person who didn't see the photograph, at least at first, was my girlfriend, Erin. When she hugged us on mile 18, she was on her expected pace of nine minutes a mile. That would have put her at the finish line just before the bombing.

But she started feeling intense knee pain near the top of Heartbreak Hill. For a while she walked, feeling an ice-pick-like stabbing in her knee with every step. She got emotional, she says, at the thought of not finishing the race. She even cried a little. But she kept pushing, until the pain subsided enough for her to jog again.

Then she ran into a wall at around mile 25, right before the overpass on Beacon Street. I don't mean a wall of pain, but a wall of runners crammed so tightly together that no one could move forward. Erin thought at first there were just too many people trying to reach the finish line. She thought the race was poorly organized, and she worried about her finishing time. Then the rumors started to filter back from the front.

The course was closed.

There had been an explosion.

No, there had been a bomb.

The bomb was near the finish line.

No, it was in the *crowd* at the finish line.

Nobody knew how many people had been hurt. No one knew if people had been killed. There was nobody giving out information. Almost every runner had someone waiting for them, but hardly anyone had a cell phone. Who would carry a cell phone while running a marathon?

Shock started to set in. People were breaking down. The woman beside Erin collapsed; Erin stayed to help her, until a nurse arrived.

Then she started to walk. Everyone else did the same: they just walked off the course. She thought of Remy, Michele, and me at the finish line. Her younger sister, Jill, was supposed to meet us there. Erin didn't know that Jill hadn't found us.

For some reason, Erin was especially worried about Remy, her best friend since middle school. She had a bad feeling something had happened to Remy. She didn't realize she was crying until a nice couple stopped and asked if she was okay. They bought her a bottle of water and let her use their cell phone. She tried Remy, then Michele, then me. No answers.

She reached her older sister, Gail, who told her two bombs had gone off in the crowd. Her little sister had seen it, but she wasn't hurt. She was across the street. She had heard Remy was hurt, but she didn't know anything else.

Erin started to panic. Something terrible had happened. People had died. Her friends were there—they were there to see her, she had asked them to be there—and at least one of them was hurt. But she couldn't do anything for her. She had no money, no cell phone, and no way to get home.

For a while, she wandered, unsure what to do. It was strangely quiet. She tried to walk to her gym, where we had agreed to meet if we missed each other in the crowd, but the road was closed. Cops were blocking the intersections leading downtown. She must have been shivering, because someone gave her a blanket. She walked for a while with a young man about her age, who couldn't reach his friends, either.

Someone saw her in her marathon number and yelled, "Congratulations. Way to go!" She realized that people going one way knew what had happened, and many of them were crying, but people coming from the other direction had no idea.

She stopped outside the Christian Science Center on Massachusetts Avenue. The streets were full of people, but eerily subdued. She thought about walking home, but it was too far. Her office at Brigham and Women's Hospital was only two miles away, though, and eventually she found herself walking that way. She didn't get to her office until almost five o'clock, two hours after the bomb went off, and six hours after she started the marathon.

The hospital was on lockdown, and she didn't have her identification card. The guards wouldn't let her in until a colleague finally noticed her. Then Jill arrived; she had walked from the finish line to the hospital, hoping to find Erin.

They took a cab to Jill's apartment and started making calls. Erin found out Michele was in emergency surgery, but Remy was stable. She couldn't find out anything about me. For some reason, she wasn't worried. She knew we must have been close to the bomb. But if Remy was only injured, she reasoned, I must be fine.

Her friend Ashley called. "Jeff's hurt," she said. "His picture is on the home page of the NPR website right now."

Erin went to the website. It was the cropped photo that didn't show my legs. I think Erin was in shock. Her mind wouldn't accept that anything terrible had happened. He's alert, she told herself. That means he's okay.

Then Courtney, a friend of Remy's whom Erin barely knew, called her.

"Remy's okay," Erin told her. "She was near the bomb, and she's in the hospital, but she's okay. Michele was hurt, too. I haven't heard from Jeff, but I'm sure he's all right."

"Jeff's not all right," Courtney said. "He lost his legs."

When her sister Gail called a few minutes later, Erin was sobbing. She had seen the uncropped photograph. "They were there for me," she said. "This is my fault."

"It's not your fault."

"I wanted Jeff to be there. I told him it was important to me. Now he has no legs."

"It's not your fault, Erin. Someone evil did this."

"You have to find him, Gail. If you find him, you have to call me."

Soon after, Big D called and told her I was at Boston Medical Center. Jill's boyfriend, Alex, drove her to the hospital. Nobody was out. The streets were deserted, except for cops. Erin didn't know it, but even the bombing site was quiet. The bodies were still on the street—they had to be examined—but everything immaterial was gone. The chief of police, Ed Davis, had learned that lesson at bombing sites in London and Israel: clean up fast. In Israel, buildings were often repaired within hours. It's a message to the terrorists: You can't stop us. We will go on.

To Erin's surprise, even Boston Medical Center was quiet. The surrounding block was closed; the guard directed her to a house across the street. There were social workers, a table of refreshments, and a checklist of victims. Someone on staff started to tell Erin what had happened to me. She told them to stop; she wanted to wait until my family arrived.

They're going to hate me, she thought. This is my fault.

Eventually, they started calling names of victims. If you were there for that person, you would trek into a side room, where a doctor would explain their condition.

There were about twenty people there for me, mostly family, when the doctors gave them the news. "He's alive."

Thank God, Erin thought.

"But we had to amputate both his legs."

The air went out of the room. People cried and hugged each other. They hugged Erin. Mom cried on her shoulder. "I'm sorry," Erin whispered. Nobody else spoke. Not even Uncle Bob, whom you usually can't pay to shut up. They had seen the photograph, and they'd known it was hopeless, but still they had been hoping.

The nurses took everyone to the intensive care unit, where I was recovering from surgery. They let Mom and Dad into my room right away. They both have since told me how terrible I looked: black eyes, cuts on my face. Both my eardrums were ruptured, and blood was seeping out of my ears. I had second-degree burns over most of my back, and lesser burns around my right eye. The heat had been so intense that my eyelashes had burned off. I had a breathing tube and bandages, and fluids running into both of my arms. They hated looking at the blanket, where the shape of my body stopped too soon. It was the worst thing they could imagine.

Until around midnight, when my blood pressure dropped and my body started to swell. The doctors said it was probably internal bleeding, that my organs must have been damaged by the blast. They rushed me into surgery. It was supposed to last an hour, but the procedure dragged, and everyone thought the worst. Why else would an hour-long surgery last two? And then three?

He must be fighting for his life.

But he isn't dead. If he was dead, they would have told us by now.

Jeff's a fighter.

Jeff's going to make it.

He would never quit on us.

Suddenly, losing my legs didn't seem so devastating. There was something much worse, and everyone was confronting it now.

Eventually, the doctors gave them the good news: My organs were fine. There was no internal bleeding. My body had been retaining fluid as a result of the blunt force trauma of the bomb blast. They had successfully drained the fluid, and I was recovering. The worst was behind me, the doctors said. I was going to live.

Everyone started to cry, even my cousin Derek. At least that was what I heard afterward, because I've never seen Derek with tears in his eyes, except when the Red Sox won the World Series in 2004. You cried for me, right, Big D?

"We still have him," Mom said, hugging the whole room. "We still have him."

I don't know what happened after that, but it was four in the morning, so I assume everyone went to sleep.

4.

By Tuesday, Boston had settled into the subdued state it would maintain for the rest of the week. Traffic was light. Conversations were slow. It was as if the city was trying to both process what had happened and respect the magnitude of the event. The night of the bombing three Emerson College students had created blue T-shirts with bright yellow letters on the front: Boston Strong. Already, the idea was starting to spread, but on Tuesday it was still too soon. The bombers had escaped, and as the day wore on, it became increasingly clear the police didn't know who they were. People weren't afraid—not in this city—but they were looking over their shoulders and doing double takes at cardboard boxes. A makeshift shrine had started on Copley Square, two blocks from the bombing site. Across the street, people covered a metal fence with running shoes. They tied small strips of cloth to the fence outside Trinity Church as symbols of peace. Within hours, there were hundreds of white strips fluttering in the spring breeze. Three different people told me the same thing: "Nobody honked, Jeff, not the entire week." In this city, that was a miracle.

At Boston Medical Center, the mood was different. With no suspects to pursue, the press turned to the victims. There were satellite trucks parked outside and reporters lurking in the lobby. After my second surgery, Erin's family had taken her back to her apartment to rest, but she had been unable to eat or sleep. She was home for only a few hours before leaving to spend the morning with Michele. The doctors had thought Michele would lose a leg, but they were optimistic emergency surgery had saved it.

Then she visited Remy, who was being treated for a large shrap-nel wound at Faulkner Hospital. By the time Erin arrived at Boston Medical Center, she couldn't walk. She had run a marathon, walked an extra five miles, and gone a day and a half without eating or sleeping. She was stressed out, traumatized, and racked with guilt. Her body gave out. Her sister Gail and her mom had to carry her up the stairs in the parking garage.

"Who are you?" the reporters shouted when they saw her limp-ing toward the doors. "Who are you here to see? Can you give us a statement?"

The intensive care area wasn't much better. Dozens of victims had been transported to BMC, many in critical condition, and relatives were still arriving from cities outside New England. The ICU was like an airport where all the flights have been canceled, and people are angry and on edge, checking their cell phones, sleeping in corners, or sitting up in chairs. There was kindness and sympathy among the families, a feeling of love brought on by being in this together, but it was edged with suspicion. Although they were not allowed, reporters had infiltrated the lounge in the ICU, so the hospital had started using false names to stop media leaks. I was "X North." I have no idea why. Most of the other victims were named after cars. Michele, who was at another hospital, was "Porsche." Porsche!

Now *that's* a secret identity.

But the leaks kept coming. By then, I had been identified as the "man in the wheelchair with no legs," and everyone in my family was receiv-ing calls. Even my friends and Erin's family had been tracked down and asked for a statement.

My family wasn't sure what to do. Should they talk about me with the press? Should they talk with the press about themselves? The world had seen the photograph. Did that mean they were entitled to infor-mation? Would it be easier to make an official statement? Or had my family already shared enough? Everyone from the *Lowell Sun*, our local newspaper, to Matt Lauer and Anderson Cooper were calling. Everyone wanted to know how the legless man in the photograph was doing.

And how *was* I doing, anyway?

That was the most troubling question. I hadn't been conscious since they anesthetized me on the operating table. I had called out for Erin once, in delirium, but otherwise I hadn't said or done anything. The doctors didn't know what to expect when I woke up, but they were pretty sure of one thing: I wouldn't remember what had happened. The blast had been so concussive, and the trauma to my body so devastating, that even if my memories survived, it would be weeks before my conscious mind could confront them and piece them back together.

I wouldn't know I had been in a bombing.

Which meant I wouldn't know I had lost my legs.

Somebody would have to tell me, and neither Mom nor Dad were up for it. Mom was almost catatonic with grief. Whenever she went in my room, her whole body shook with crying. Erin told me she hardly spoke, except to occasionally ask, "How? How could this happen to us?"

"I don't know," Erin would tell her. "But it did. So we have to face it."

My dad had swung the other way. He was almost manic: yelling at the nurses, angry at the doctors for not saving my legs. It wasn't long before he was arguing with Aunt Jenn, who had taken on the role of Mom's protector and voice, and both of them were expecting Erin to side with them.

They argued about the media. My dad had granted a few interviews, not so much out of desire to be published, I think, but from an inability to stop talking. Mom wasn't happy. "Who is he to talk about Jeff?" she said.

Only my dad, Mom.

"I think we should keep the drama to a minimum," Erin said.

They argued about the donations. Two strangers in Colorado had set up a Facebook page in my honor, and donations were rolling in. Two friends at Costco, Jon and Aubrie Park, had created "Bauman Strong" bracelets and were selling them for $1. They had expected to sell a few hundred, but thousands had already been sold.

"It's Jeff's money," Erin said, "so it's his decision what to do with it."

They argued about where I would live after I got out of the hospital.

"He's not even conscious yet," Erin said in exasperation. "We need to focus on what Jeff needs now, when he wakes up, not what he needs a month from now."

In the end, it was decided that Erin should tell me what had happened. She was the one person I had called out for. Everyone knew how much I cared for and trusted her. And besides, she was the only neutral party.

I know it was a burden, but knowing Erin, she shouldered it without complaint. At least my family hadn't rejected or blamed her, like she had feared. She stayed with me for several hours that day, although it couldn't have been easy, either in her condition or mine. Erin was exhausted and overwhelmed. I was so bruised and burned I didn't look like myself, and my body was... short. Everyone was worried about my mental state.

"If Jeff can do this with me," Erin had told her sister Jill the previous night, when they were down in the hospital lobby taking a break, "then I can handle anything. But he has to want it. I can't do it for him."

How would I react when I woke up and discovered what had happened? Would I fall into despair? Would I be angry? Would I even be myself anymore?

Around five that evening, Erin decided to leave. Michele was awake and recovering from another surgery, so Erin and Gail drove across town to spend a few hours with her.

And of course, that was exactly when I decided to wake up.

5.

The first thing I remember is my best friend Sully's face. He was standing beside the bed, looking down at me. I turned and saw his ex-girlfriend Jill standing on the other side. Honestly, they didn't look so good.

It was late afternoon on Tuesday, almost thirty hours after the bombing. According to the doctors, I wasn't expected to be awake until Wednesday. So of course Sully takes credit.

"I shouted, 'BAU-MAN, wake up,'" he tells people proudly, especially after he's had a few. "I barked it, just like that: 'BO-MAN! BO-MAN! Wake up!' And he woke up."

What actually woke me up was Jill stroking my hair. I was lying somewhere, and I felt something lightly touching my head, and I opened my eyes.

My whole body hurt. They had me on morphine for the worst of the pain, but it still felt like I'd taken one of those movie beatings, where the bad guys kick you a few extra times in the stomach for good measure, even after you're down. When I turned my head, it hurt. I couldn't even gather my thoughts, I was in so much pain.

I tried to swallow, but I couldn't. My throat was dry, but I couldn't move my tongue. I panicked. I thought I was choking. Then I noticed the tube jammed down my throat.

I stared at Sully and Jill. They were staring at me. Waiting. What could I say? Nothing, not with that tube in my mouth. I lifted my arm and made a motion like writing. I think it was Jill who gave me the pencil and pad of paper.

I wrote: *Lt. Dan.*

Sully laughed out loud. "Only Bauman," he said. Lt. Dan was For-
rest Gump's commanding officer. He lost his legs in Vietnam.

I motioned toward the lower part of my body.

"Yeah," Sully said sadly. "You lost your legs."

I motioned for the paper again. I had one more thing to say. I
wrote...

Oh man, I wish I knew what I had written, because everybody
remembers something different. It's been reported many times, first
by Bloomberg News, then by the *Boston Globe* and others, that I wrote
Bag. Saw the guy. Looked right at me. That's what Chris—my half brother
on Dad's side—remembers, and he's the one who talked to the press.
The family members on Mom's side disagree. They say I drew pictures,
although they can't agree on what I drew.

Sully remembers me pointing to my eyes. Then drawing a backpack. A bomb. Then a face. I gave the *saw it* sign again with my fingers.

And he understood.

He walked out into the hallway with my note, his hands shaking.
That's the one detail everyone agrees on: that when Sully came out
of my room, he was white and shaking. He didn't say a word. He just
handed my note to Uncle Bob (or, in some versions, to my dad). My
family had just come out of a meeting with the FBI liaison for victim
relations, an ass-kicking older woman named Renee Morell, who had
been explaining how the FBI would help relatives with hotel rooms
and meal credits.

Uncle Bob (or maybe my dad) passed the note to Ms. Morell, who
called the local FBI office. Or maybe Uncle Bob called the FBI, whose
number was posted in the hallway.

Until recently, I had assumed the agents were simply waiting for
me. I told the EMT in the ambulance that I had seen the bomber, and
for me, that seemed like only seconds ago. Surely, I thought, someone
would be waiting to take my testimony. That was why it took them
only a minute to arrive.

I found out later it took almost an hour, I just don't remember it. In fact, I don't even remember writing the note. I remember writing "Lt. Dan," and watching Sully's face turn from fear to laughter, and feeling...good. Like myself. Then my breathing tube was out, and two FBI agents and the commissioner of the Massachusetts State Police were standing beside my bed. They pulled the curtain behind them, *Law & Order* style, pulled up some chairs, and started asking questions.

They asked me what I had seen.

"I saw the guy."

They asked me for a description.

Dark baseball cap. Dark jacket, maybe leather. Dark sunglasses.

"What kind?"

Um...aviators.

His jacket was open. He was wearing a gray shirt. And a backpack. It was a JanSport.

"A JanSport? You remember that?"

Clearly.

They asked me for a physical description.

Taller than me. Stubble. Light skin.

"He was white?"

Yes, white.

Why did you notice him?

"He was all business."

That was the first time I said that, but it sticks with me now. It's the phrase that jumps into my mind whenever I picture Tamerlan Tsarnaev. He was a bad dude. Not bad like cool, but bad like angry. Troubled. One look, and you knew he was not someone to mess with. He'd punch your teeth out just for bumping him. He was all business.

"He wasn't there to enjoy himself," I told the FBI. "He was there for a reason."

I told them how we eyeballed each other, and then how he was gone, but his backpack was still there, on the ground. The JanSport.

"Just look for me," I said. "If you have video, look for me. He was beside me. Right beside me."

At the end, I wrote down a description. That's all I know for sure. I think the conversation happened the way I described it. I remember all those things. I can picture them right now. But is that exactly what I told the FBI? How can I know for sure? I don't think they recorded the conversation, and I don't know what happened to my written description or my original note. I assume it's all in their case files somewhere.

"Thank you," one of the agents said at the end. "Do you mind if we come back later?"

I nodded, and they left. At that point, I was wiped out. But I was happy. I'd done as much as I could do, and it felt good, like I was part of the team. I turned to my dad, who had been sitting quietly in the corner. "Do you think I helped?"

"You helped," he said. "Before they talked to you, I don't think they had any idea who they were looking for."

That didn't make any sense to me. This guy had been standing in a crowd. There were cameras everywhere. How could they not know who he was? How could I have been the only one to notice him?

My brother Tim said later that he overheard the FBI agents talking by the elevator on their way out.

"What do you think?" one of them said. "The kid's on a lot of painkillers."

"It's the best information we've got," the other replied.

The agents came back a few hours later. This time, they brought a stack of photographs. It was late at night, and the hospital was quiet. I sat in bed with a flashlight for twenty minutes, studying each face. I handed them back. None of them were the guy I had seen. If the agents were disappointed, they didn't show it.

"I want to see Erin," I said after they left.

Erin had just arrived at Michele's room when she got the call that I was alert. By the time she'd made it back, the FBI was interviewing me. Then my family had wanted to see me. Then the FBI had come back again.

It was around midnight before we finally got time to ourselves. Erin's sister Gail remembers looking in the doorway window and seeing us sitting on the bed, whispering, our heads close together. There were two security guards stationed outside my door, but otherwise the hospital was still, until a nurse came by to check on me.

"Can you give them a minute?" Gail asked.

She did. The nurse left us sitting together, under a single small light, with my cords and tubes dangling around us. I don't know what I said. I had been blown up; Erin had been without basic comforts for two days. I hope that I said, "I love you."

I probably said, "Thank you for being here."

There was no place I'd rather have been. That was what Erin told me later. She said that when she saw me smile, she knew I was still her person. And she knew this was where she wanted to be. With me.

———

I didn't sleep that night, so I was awake when the FBI agents arrived early on Wednesday morning. Again, they gave me a stack of photographs without explanation. Again, I studied every face. None looked like the guy I had seen, and only a few fit my general description. I think they were looking for accomplices. They wanted to know if I had noticed any of these people in the crowd. I told them I hadn't. The guy had been alone.

"We'd like to bring in a sketch artist," they said.

"Sure," I replied.

"But only after his surgery," a nurse added.

The original amputation of my legs had been an emergency procedure. They chopped through my knees and sealed the wounds to save my life. Now I needed a formal amputation to even my legs and shape my stumps for prosthetics. Legs the same length would mean the same amount of work on both sides. Over time, this would help prevent back and hip pain, common problems for people with artificial legs. The better this surgery went, explained my surgeon, Dr. Jeffrey Kalish, the easier it would be for me to walk again.

And that was all I wanted. I wanted to walk.

The surgery took several hours, as Dr. Kalish separated each layer of skin, tissue, and muscle in my legs. He cut each layer a little shorter than the one beside it, angling inward with the outer layers longest. Lastly, he sawed off the ends of my femurs and tucked the muscles, then the arteries, then my fatty tissues and nerves, around them. My skin came last, pulled together at the ends to encase everything inside. Like a sausage. When I woke up that afternoon, I was four inches shorter, and my legs were on fire. Bloody bandages were wrapped around the ends, but there were no stitches. The wounds would be left open for a few days, so that blood and fluid could drain.

When the FBI sketch artist arrived soon after, the nurses weren't happy.

"It's up to Jeff," they told the FBI while glancing at me, clearly trying to convince me to send them away. They wanted to catch the bombers as much as anyone, but I was in a delicate condition. I had just woken up from major surgery. I had bleeding wounds. I was susceptible to infections, infarctions, and a hundred other types of medical-sounding stuff.

I hate medical-sounding stuff.

But I wanted to work with the sketch artist. I wanted to do my part. We went over it again and again: talking, erasing, drawing. Stopping while I tried to picture the face of the killer, the guy who stared at me, all business, secretly excited by the fact that he was taking my life. It took two hours, but in the end, I was amazed. The drawing looked exactly like the guy who had stood beside me.

That evening, the press later reported, the police found a suspect in store surveillance video taken near the scene, along with a possible accomplice. My description was essential, they said, because FBI experts had been sifting through hundreds of hours of footage, featuring thousands of faces. It was vital to narrow the focus.

I don't know if that's true. I don't know how much I really helped, because the FBI agents never came back. I meet with the FBI every month, just like many other victims, so they can fill me in on the case, and ask me a few questions if needed, but they don't tell me much.

I talk with state and local cops all the time, though. I meet them at charity events, or they come over and shake my hand when I'm out.

"We heard about what you did," they tell me. "Identifying those guys."

"It was nothing," I say. "Just trying to do my part."

"No, Jeff," they tell me. "It wasn't nothing." Sometimes I feel like they want to tell me more, but they can't. I understand. It's an ongoing investigation. It's strictly need-to-know, and I'm a civilian. I don't have a need. "You should be proud," they tell me. "You're a big part of this. You got the ball rolling."

"Okay, okay," I say, laughing. "But you guys are the heroes. You nailed them."

"No," they always say. "We're not heroes. We were just doing our jobs."

6.

People always want to know how I felt in those first few days. Was I guilty that I hadn't done more to stop the bombing? Was I angry? Was I afraid? Was I Boston Strong?

No, I was happy to be alive.

Besides that, I was in pain. It was intense physical pain, the kind that doesn't leave you much energy for anything else. It was kind of like when you really have to go to the bathroom, I mean, like a real emergency, when you think you might not make it. You can't focus on anything else, right?

My pain was like that. The hospital had me on a four-hour cycle of pain medication, but even when the pills were at their strongest, I hurt. Everywhere. My arm where shrapnel had punctured it, my stomach where they had sliced me open for surgery. With both my eardrums ruptured, my head was always ringing. The burns on my back were so raw, it was uncomfortable to lie on them, but even more uncomfortable to move. I couldn't yet roll onto my side, but every time I moved even a few inches, it felt like my skin was sliding off.

And every time my legs touched anything—the sheets, my IV tubes, each other—pain shot through my body. The nerves in my legs were lit up by the blast, and they were ready to fire. Mostly the pain was sharp, like needles, but sometimes it would increase without warning, until it felt like someone was pounding the ends of my legs with a baseball bat. Coffee would cramp my legs, so I only drank it once in the hospital. Certain sounds and smells would set off convulsions in my thighs, sending pain cascading through my torso and down into my phantom limbs.

I tried to ignore it. I had a morphine button I could push, but I tried not to use it. I talked with my family. I tried to watch the news, but all they talked about was the bombing. And every time they talked about the bombing, sooner or later, they'd show pictures of explosions and blood, and they'd show that photograph of me in the wheelchair.

So I watched a lot of ESPN, drowning the hours in scores and highlights. It was late in the hockey season, but early for baseball. The Red Sox were in Cleveland. I watched as Victorino slapped in a few runs, and Aceves melted down in the sixth, but I was watching from a different planet. I was on a lot of medication; I felt best when the world just floated past.

I knew I needed to stay positive, especially around Mom. That was my priority. Mom had always struggled. She had worried about me all my life, even when I was a little kid. I didn't have to see her red eyes and drawn face to know this was killing her. So I never told her about my pain. I called her in right after taking my medicine, so I was less likely to wince or have a panic attack. I tried not to complain.

"I knew there were two ways you could go," Mom tells me now, her hands still shaking. "You could be..." She stops. Mom doesn't say *depressed*, because she doesn't like that word, but that's what she means. "You could have taken it hard, Jeff. Or you could be Bauman."

That's her nickname for me. Mom calls me Bauman or Bo. Jeff is my dad's name.

"I don't know if you remember..."

"I don't, Mom," I tell her, knowing what's coming.

"...we were all standing over you."

"I know. It's creepy."

"And you opened your eyes. This was early, maybe Tuesday, so we weren't expecting it. We didn't know what to say. Your eyes went from one person to the next, and nobody was sure whether you recognized them or not. Finally, you tried to speak. But you couldn't. So it must have been Tuesday, right? Anyway, I bent down so you could whisper in my ear.

" 'What is this,' you whispered, 'a funeral viewing? Everybody sit down.' "

Mom usually cries when she tells that story. I've heard it five times, and maybe four of those times she's ended in tears. That's how important it is to her.

"That's when I knew," she says. "You were still my Jeffrey. You weren't going to be ... sad. You were Bauman strong."

I'm not sure about Mom's story. There are certain parts of it that don't quite work. I was in the emergency intensive care unit, for one thing, so only two people were allowed in my room at a time. I know my family constantly broke that rule (we aren't the best at following rules), but how could the whole family have been there?

And when I woke up, I was on a breathing tube. How could I have whispered even those two sentences to her?

But that doesn't mean I don't believe her. In fact, I know it's true, that the moment *must* have happened, because it means so much to her. I know Mom. I know how her worry would have crushed her. She cries now, listing the things I can't do: play hockey (I quit playing when I was thirteen), ride a bicycle (I don't even own one), run a marathon (that was never gonna happen). I can imagine how she felt, worrying that I would never smile and be happy again.

And besides, my brother Tim tells a similar story. In his version, everyone was there, and he was squeezing my hand, asking if I knew who he was, when I made the joke.

So maybe it happened on Wednesday, after my third surgery. Or maybe it happened on Monday night, before my second surgery. Maybe they had me off the breathing tube for a while, before slicing open my stomach and poking around inside me.

It doesn't matter to me. It doesn't matter if it never quite happened like that. Everybody has a story about those days, which they swear is true, even though none of the stories are the same. They say it happened on Tuesday, while someone else swears it was the next week.

Or they say, "I remember, because I was there," when someone else knows for certain, for *certain*, that he was the only one in my room.

I don't remember my funeral visitation joke, but it feels right, because that was exactly how I tried to be: the same Jeff. Happy-go-lucky. Smiling. Making a joke out of everything, even the worst of things.

It was hard. Mom fidgeted whenever she was in my room, like she didn't know what to do with herself. Like she was scared to be around me. Aunt Jenn did most of the talking. Mom stood in the background, staring at me, in a way that said both *I love you more than anything* and *I am so sad when I look at you.*

She felt sorry for me. I didn't want anyone to feel sorry for me.

And she kept asking me how I was doing.

I hated that question.

What did she want me to say? *I love it here! I'm doing swell!*

Most of my relatives were like that. They were too attentive: asking me if I was all right every time I winced, wondering what they could do for me. Even my brother Tim treated me like an invalid.

"Jeff, you all right, bro? Want me to call the nurse? How about some water? Does your leg hurt?"

Yes, jerk-face, my leg hurts! My legs feel like Popsicle sticks some asshole kid snapped in half.

It was better with Erin. With Erin, I didn't feel any pressure. We could sit in the room together, barely talking, and be happy.

I never doubted her. We had been together for only a year. Less than a month before the bombing, we had broken up. She would never have just left me lying in the hospital, but she could have drifted away. She liked routine. She had a plan for her life. A legless boyfriend who needed her for emotional and practical support—who else was going to adjust my hospital gown?—was never in her plans.

Yet the first thing I did, whenever I woke up, was ask for Erin.

And she was there.

It was Erin who told me the investigation was stalled. She told me about the media crush. She told me that as soon as they walked outside the hospital, reporters were shoving cameras in her face. A British television show had lifted a picture of her and me together from her Facebook page. Now every station was showing it. It was the standard "before" picture of the legless man.

"Your dad keeps talking to the press," Erin said sadly. I think she had this idea that, if we all stayed quiet, the attention would go away.

"It's his decision," I said.

She told me about other families in the intensive care unit, like the Odoms, who were from California. Mr. Odom's son-in-law played for the Revolution, Boston's professional soccer team. His daughter had been running in the marathon. His wife survived the bombing untouched, but a large piece of shrapnel had almost severed Mr. Odom's leg at the hip. His wife and daughter had been at the hospital with him ever since.

"Gail went to run an errand to the drugstore for Mrs. Odom," Erin told me. "Mr. Odom is on life support. She never expected to be in town this long."

That information made me uncomfortable, even more than my legs. I didn't like thinking about the larger situation—all the death and destruction. I didn't know what to say.

"You've got an afro," Erin said, patting my hair.

"You're joking," I said.

"It's true."

"Give me a mirror."

She did. I couldn't believe how beat up I looked. A Jason Statham–type roundhouse kick to the right eye. Burns on my forehead. The heat of the blast had singed my hair, making it stick out in all directions. "I think it looks good, E," I said. "I think I should keep this hair. How high do you think it will grow?"

It really did look good, by the way. I think Erin agreed that I was handsome, despite my black eye. "It will be nice when your eyebrows grow back," she said.

"Afro eyebrows! Do you think it could happen?"

She touched my left arm, the only part of my body that didn't hurt. She put her head close to mine and whispered, "I'm sorry."

"Don't say that," I told her.

She turned off the light and hugged me. "Watch the legs," I said.

I put my arm around her. She was quiet for a long time. I could feel her breathing so slowly that I thought she might have gone to sleep. Neither of us had taken a shower since the bombing, and I'm not sure either of us had slept.

"You're famous, you know," she said finally.

"I don't want to be famous for this."

She sighed. "That's what I thought." I've said before how different Erin and I were, but in the important ways, we were the same.

She kissed me on the forehead. My legs were throbbing. "I just want to be left alone," I said.

But then I thought: No, not alone. I want to be with you.

7.

Thursday, April 18, will be remembered in Boston as the day the manhunt began. It might become a new holiday now, part of the legend of Patriot's Day, along with the marathon and Paul Revere's ride and the battle at the Old North Bridge. At least for a few years, anyway, until the memory starts to fade.

But Thursday didn't start that way, at least for me. It started with a homemade Pop-Tart.

While I was in surgery on Wednesday, my store manager at Costco, Kevin "Heavy Kevy" Horst, had arrived at the hospital with a care package and a stack of paperwork. Mom met him in the lobby, flanked by her sisters, Aunt Jenn and Aunt Karen. After the media blitz on Tuesday, the hospital wasn't letting anyone without a pass through to the ICU.

Kevin sat with them and explained my benefits: disability, the Employee Assistance Program, the "dismemberment" benefit in the insurance package.

I was fortunate. Costco's health insurance was top-notch. I'm more fortunate than many of my fellow victims, who are struggling not just with bills, but with insurers who don't want to pay for their long recoveries, or the lifetime of health issues many of us will endure. Someone told me later that investors had been hammering Costco for years over its health insurance policies, insisting they offer a less expensive (and far worse) plan. I guess that was worth a few pennies on the stock price. Costco always said no.

A year ago, I couldn't have cared less. In fact, a few months before the bombing, I had tried to quit the insurance program. I was young and healthy, and I figured I'd be healthy for years. I never even went to the doctor for checkups. Why did I need to pay out of pocket every week for something I wasn't even using? A hundred bucks a month could come in very handy.

My department manager, Maya, talked me out of it. "It's important," she told me. "You may not understand that now, but someday you will."

I figured it wasn't worth arguing about, so I dropped the idea. That turned out to be the greatest decision I never made. Even with good insurance, my medical bills are high. My artificial legs cost $100,000 each, and my insurance paid only half. I was fortunate that several charities, like Wiggle Your Toes, which provides limbs for recent amputees, covered the initial cost. But what about when the legs wear out? Or when they need repairs? Or when I suffer complications next year, or the year after that, from the trauma to my body? If I had to guess, I'd say I have a million dollars in medical bills ahead of me.

That's one of the reasons I'm so thankful to everyone who has donated to me. I try not to think about the future, but Mom thinks about it all the time. You saved her from a lifetime of worry.

"Thank you," Mom told Kevin, when Aunt Jenn finally stopped asking him questions. "Thank you. I had no idea he was so well taken care of."

Kevin then started ticking off other things he had set up for them. The hospital parking deck was expensive, so Kevin had wrangled three free parking spaces for my family less than a block away. His gym had provided free passes so my family could have a place to exercise or relax. He had gone to local restaurants and asked, "If I buy gift cards for Jeff's family, will you match the amount?"

"No," the restaurants said, "we'll give you as many gift cards as you need."

The FBI was providing hotel rooms for my close relatives, but other friends and relatives had no place in the city to stay. Kevin's friend offered her apartment for a few weeks, so they wouldn't have to drive back and forth to Chelmsford. Erin's family, who lived more than an hour away, stayed there several times.

In the middle of all this, my dad showed up in the lobby, agitated as usual. "This is all nice," he said, after listening to all Kevin had done. "But I want to know one thing: if Jeff makes it out of this, will you hire him back?"

"We can't hire him back," Kevin told him. "He still works for us. We're not going to let him go."

Dad shook Kevin's hand, then started to cry.

The next morning, Kevin showed up in my room with that Pop-Tart–like pastry. It was homemade by a nearby restaurant named Flour, which must have been Kevin's favorite, because he talked about it all the time.

"You don't have to do this," I said.

"Costco gave me time off to take care of you," Kevin told me. "It's the least I can do."

He handed me a new cell phone. It was much nicer than the old one I had lost in the bombing. The old one had been held together with tape. "From your friends at work," he said. "We all chipped in to buy it for you."

"Thank you, sir," I said, addressing him in the respectful way I always had on the job.

"Please, call me Kevin."

"Yes, sir."

Of course, that was my Thursday morning. For the rest of Boston, and maybe even the country, Thursday started with an interfaith service at the Cathedral of the Holy Cross, near the site of the bombing. This was the first official public expression of grief, and Boston turned out. By then, the city had rallied. Boston Strong was everywhere. On clothes. On the destination signs on the buses. On the front of the Museum of Fine Arts. The streets outside the cathedral were mobbed with everyone from dignitaries in formal dress to motorcycle gangs.

More than an hour before the service, the line to get in was already more than a block long.

A representative of President Barack Obama's office came to the hospital to offer a ticket to each victim's family. Mom wanted Erin to go, but she turned it down.

"Tell President Obama I'm sorry," Erin said, "but I can't handle it right now. I'm a mess."

Other family members wanted to go, but there weren't enough tickets. They would have to wait in line. Kevin wouldn't hear of that. "Don't worry," he said. "We'll take care of you."

He started making calls. Within twenty minutes, he had secured my family ten seats at the front of the church. The governor's office had authorized it. That was the first time I realized the name Jeff Bauman meant something to people in Boston, and that the city was going to take care of us.

"Thank you, sir," I told Kevin. It was an instinct. This was my boss's boss.

"Please, Jeff," he said, "you don't need to call me sir."

I watched some of the ceremony, which was carried live across the country. President Obama spoke of the victims. The city's religious leaders, of all faiths, urged peace and love to counter anger and hate. Like many others, I thought of Martin Richard, the eight-year-old boy who died in the blast. There was a famous picture of him, taken the year before, smiling (with one of his front baby teeth missing) and holding a handwritten sign that said: No more hurting people. Peace.

"It was beautiful," said Uncle Bob, who had walked to the ceremony from the hospital. "A beautiful service."

"But too soon," Aunt Cathleen added.

A few hours later, I received my first surprise visitor. Late one night, my dad had been down in the hospital lobby, working through his feelings. By which I mean he was pacing, talking to himself, and crying. By then, Massachusetts had posted state troopers at the hospital door to protect the privacy of victims. This trooper, Carlo Matromate, happened to be chatty.

"Who are you here for?" he asked.

"My son." My dad told him about me.

"How's he doing?" Carlo asked.

"He's down," my dad said. "He tries not to show it."

"Tell you what," the trooper said. "I used to work security, and I know a few Patriots. You think that would cheer him up?"

"I'm sure it would," my dad said. "Jeff loves the Patriots."

So Thursday, around noon, in walked a state trooper, escorting Julian Edelman. Now, Julian Edelman is no typical star. He went to a small college. He was a late-round draft pick. He worked his way up from punt returns, where he was the best to ever play the game. Everybody in Boston loved Julian Edelman. He was the little guy who kept fighting. He was tough.

And here he was, in my hospital room, calling me tough. Telling me to keep going, because the whole city was pulling for me.

At first, it was...wow. What do you say? But after a few minutes, it was...well, Julian Edelman was a regular dude. Just a good guy to talk to. He brought me a football, one he'd intercepted and run back for a touchdown when he filled in on defense for half a year. We were throwing it around the room when suddenly, boom, in walked Bradley Cooper.

I'm not a fan of the *Hangover* movies, but I love *Silver Linings Playbook*. My dad is a Philly guy, so I knew those characters. And now Pat Solitano was here, standing in my hospital room with his hand out, saying, "Hi, Jeff. I'm Bradley. It's an honor to meet you."

I heard later he was in town filming a movie, and he had been at the interfaith service. Afterward, he walked over to the hospital to see someone he knew, who happened to be on my floor. Somehow, Kevin found out he was there, so he waited by the elevator. For security reasons, only one elevator bank was allowed to stop on the fifth floor.

"Hi, Mr. Cooper. So nice to see you. Wow. I don't know if you've heard of Jeff Bauman. He was the man in the wheelchair. He lost both his legs in the bombing."

"Yeah, I know who he is."

"He's a fan, and I know he'd like to meet you."

"Who are you?"

"I'm, um . . . I'm his brother. He's right on this floor."

"Well, then, let's go."

So that's how I ended up tossing a football, in an intensive care hospital room, with Bradley Cooper and Julian Edelman. Julian had a picture taken with the three of us and Carlo, the state trooper. He posted it online later that day, so now the world has a copy, too.

My favorite detail in the photo is my grandma. She's in the front corner, looking toward me, like she doesn't even know a photo is being taken, even though the rest of us are posing. I'm even giving a thumbs-up. I don't get to see Grandma much, because she's my dad's mom and lives near Philly, but I love her. When she found out what had happened, she had to be there for me, *had to*, even though she no longer travels. My aunt had driven her from south Jersey the day before. I'm sure they squabbled the whole ten hours.

"Who was that?" Grandma asked, after everyone had gone.

"That was Julian Edelman and Bradley Cooper, Mom," my dad said.

"Oh." Silence. "Who are they?"

"Bradley Cooper is a movie star, Mom. He was in *Silver Linings Playbook*."

"Oh, yes, I've heard of him," she said, although she clearly hadn't. She paused. "He's handsome. I knew I should have done my hair."

I was telling Erin about that a few hours later. "I guess there's a silver lining to being famous, right, E?" I said, twirling the football.

Then I looked down at the flat place in the sheets where my legs should have been. No, I thought, this still sucks.

8.

That afternoon, most of my relatives left the hospital. There was a candlelight vigil on the Chelmsford Center common that night to honor the victims of the bombing, and my family wanted to be there.

Shortly after they left, the FBI announced a news conference for 5:00 p.m. At the news conference, they released six surveillance photographs taken on Boylston Street and asked for help identifying the men shown. Like the rest of Boston, I didn't know that was going to happen. The FBI never came back and asked me to comment on the footage. I didn't know, until that moment, that there were two suspects.

But when I saw the footage of suspect 1, even though it didn't clearly show his face, I knew they had the right guy. That backpack, that jacket. My stomach dropped. It was him.

The police commissioner, Ed Davis, later called the release of the footage "a turning point in the investigation." The city had been waiting for a way to help, and the FBI had finally given it one. The tips poured in by the thousands. A friend of Dzhokhar Tsarnaev, Tamerlan's little brother, texted him, joking that he looked like one of the suspects. Dzhokhar, who had been working out in the gym and going to his college classes like any other student all week, responded, essentially, Ha. Ha. That's funny. By the way, I'm leaving town and never coming back.

Meanwhile, the media set to work analyzing the photos as all of Boston watched. Were the suspects Middle Eastern? If so, were they Muslim? Was this a planned attack, like those in London, Madrid, and Mumbai? Were these the bag men for a larger organization? Or were they lone wolves?

And how sure was the FBI that these were the guys?

By evening, the mainstream and social media firestorm had pointed to numerous false suspects, including a student who had committed suicide weeks before (his body was later found) and, famously, on the front page of the *New York Post*, a local track coach and a high school runner. It was a natural reaction. After five days of nothing, the world was energized. Finally, there was something to talk about.

I didn't want any part of it.

"What time is the Sox game?" I asked Derek, who was staying with me for the night. I hated being alone, especially at night, when I couldn't sleep. It scared me. So two people, at least, always stayed with me.

Usually it was the younger generation: Sully, Big D, and Chris. Sometimes Erin and Gail. That night, it was Big D and my older brother, Tim. I say "brother," but Tim is technically my half brother. He came from a previous relationship, before Mom met my dad, and I didn't know him until I was twenty-one years old, when he called Mom out of the blue. Say what you will about Mom, but she's bighearted. When she knew Tim needed her, she took him in. And from that moment on, Tim and I have been close. We've been watching baseball and drinking beer together ever since.

Normal life—that's what it felt like with those guys. Put beers in our hands, and it would have been just like a hundred other nights we'd spent together. The Sox had gone into the crapper the last two years, collapsing in 2011 and missing the playoffs on the last day of the season, then firing their manager, dumping salary, and proceeding to finish dead last in 2012, with the worst record for a Boston baseball team since 1965.

They had a new manager, again, and a few new players, but nobody high profile. They'd gotten off to a hot start, sure, but nobody was expecting much. Baseball is a slow, spread-out, and rambling game, played almost every night for six months, 162 games in 182 days. Early-season baseball is full of promise and false hope. It's the perfect way to kill off a couple hours.

And that was what I wanted, especially with the bombers plastered all over the news. I just wanted to forget the nurses, who were always poking and prodding me; the sudden throbbing in my legs that made me want to scream; the unsettling sound of walking in the hallway; and the odor of the bomb, a mixture of fireworks and burning flesh, that never seemed to go away. I went to sleep that night the only way possible: to the sound of Jenny Dell working the sideline, and Tim and Big D arguing about something that happened in 2009. The Sox were leading... "Salty" Saltalamacchia homered... Uehara was out... Bailey was coming in...

I woke up like I often did, jerking upright with my heart pounding. It was dark, but a light was flickering. Big D and Tim were crowded around the television with the volume low, watching the news. There had been a shooting, a carjacking, an attempted robbery.

"It's them," I said.

"No," Big D said. "They're saying it's not related."

"It's just punks," Tim added.

But I knew it was the bombers. I knew it. I had never considered how they would be caught, but as soon as I heard that people were shooting at cops, I knew there was no other way for them to go.

Later that night, I had my first nightmare. I can't remember what it was about, but I woke up shouting for Big D.

"I'm here, Jeff. I'm here," Tim said. He was slumped in a chair by the door. "Nothing to worry about, buddy. We're here."

9.

I texted Kevin at 6:00 the next morning: U up?

He was up. Everybody was up. Social media had exploded when word of the shootout in Watertown, a suburb only a few miles from downtown, started to trickle out after midnight. Kevin had been up since 4:00 a.m., glued to his television and his e-mail account, as had most of Boston. A police officer was dead. Another was in critical condition. One suspect had died in a gun battle with police, but the second had escaped. It was believed he was hiding somewhere in Watertown, although Cambridge was also on lockdown. The suspect had driven to Watertown from Cambridge in a stolen car.

"We believe this to be a terrorist," Police Commissioner Ed Davis told reporters about 4:30 a.m. Friday. "We believe this to be a man who came here to kill people."

Pop-Tart? I texted Kevin.

Kevin showed up within half an hour with several boxes of treats for everyone. Flour wasn't opening that day, given the situation in the city, but the bakery had already finished the morning pastries. The assistant manager had given Kevin as much as he could carry.

Kevin stayed that morning and chatted, while we kept one eye on the news. I think he was trying to keep my mind off the manhunt. We talked about music, I remember, something we'd often discussed at the store. I told him I loved Bob Dylan and Radiohead. He knew I played guitar, so he asked about James Taylor. James Taylor lived in Massachusetts.

"Erin loves James Taylor," I said. "The original JT."

When Uncle Bob and his kids arrived, Kevin went home.

Thank you, sir, I texted him.

Not long after, the FBI released a photograph of the second suspect: Dzhokhar Tsarnaev. Suddenly, after five days of waiting, Boston was looking at the face of evil, the person who had stuffed ball bearings into pressure cookers with the intention of ripping people apart. I don't know what the rest of Boston thought. After five days, it was stunning to see him so clearly, right in front of us. For a while, nobody spoke.

"Shit," Big D said finally. "He's a kid."

It wasn't too long before the media got hold of a photo of the other suspect: his older brother, Tamerlan.

"That's him," I said as soon as I saw it.

There wasn't much more to say. Tamerlan Tsarnaev had blown my legs off. He was the one. Now he was dead, and his brother was cornered. I thought I'd feel happy, but I just felt numb.

"Turn the channel," I said. "Let's watch something else."

Then Erin called Tim. She was with Gail and her friend Ashley in her apartment in Brighton, just across the Charles River from Watertown.

"They're saying Jeff identified the bombers," she said. "That he was the only one who saw them. What if the brother comes after Jeff? He's desperate. He knows I'm Jeff's girlfriend. It's been on the news. What if he comes after me?"

Erin admits now that she was paranoid. That it didn't make sense for Dzhokhar to come after her. But in those first hours, with one police officer dead and another critically wounded, anything seemed possible. It didn't seem crazy for Erin to feel like a target, because as much as I tried to deny my fear, I felt like a target, too, and I was in a secure hospital with two security guards outside my door.

Nobody was supposed to know I had helped the FBI. My family had all agreed that was information we would never reveal. Without legs, I felt vulnerable. And who knew how deep this plot went? The press was reporting two suspects, but what if they were part of a larger group? What if they had friends?

They were stupid kids. Who put them up to this? Tamerlan was a psychopath, sure, but who taught him how to kill?

I'm still not convinced, even today, that they acted alone. Betty Crocker Bomb Making, that's what they call this kind of attack. Get a recipe off the Internet, make a bomb. It happened that way in London and Madrid. It happens that way in Iraq and Afghanistan all the time.

But it wasn't quite that simple. The bomb that blew off my legs was detonated by the control panel of a remote control car. The part from the car was in the bomb; Dzhokhar had the control. It was the only piece, the FBI told me, that the bombers couldn't have manufactured themselves. They found the person who modified the controller. He was somewhere on the West Coast. He said he didn't know what the remote would be used for, and I guess that's possible.

But it still makes me uncomfortable, like maybe this was bigger than we know.

And if it wasn't, if any idiot can make a bomb, is that any better? That only means it's easier for imitators.

So I wish, I really wish, that Chris hadn't leaked the news of my involvement.

I don't blame Chris. I love the kid. He says he didn't know the two women he was talking with were reporters, that he just met them outside the hospital and started talking. Chris is my younger brother; he looked up to me. He was strong. He was one of my boys.

He had never experienced tragedy before. I knew he was exhausted and upset. I remember trying to make him laugh. I'd pull on my oxygen mask, breathe deeply, and say in my best Darth Vader voice: "Chris, I am your father. Now get your daddy a cheeseburger and fries." Chris was supposed to be with me at the marathon, but I had invited him too late. He couldn't get the day off from his job at McDonald's. He had this idea that he could have changed things if he'd been there. That's how you think when you're twenty-two.

So he slipped up, and an article claiming I had identified the suspects (really only partly accurate) appeared on Bloomberg News that morning. This was the middle of the manhunt, and everyone—everyone—picked up and repeated the news. We turned to a news channel after Erin called, and my face was in continuous rotation. Bauman. No legs. Jeff Bauman. Identified the bombers. Tsarnaev. Bauman. Tsarnaev. They kept showing the photo of Erin and me that had been pulled off Facebook. Bauman the hero. Bauman and his girlfriend. Did we mention he lost his legs?

Erin called back half an hour later, while Tim was on hold with the Brighton police. She had talked with an FBI agent who told her not to worry—the bomber was on the run, and she was in no danger. She called her father, who told her to stay put, he was on his way. She sounded better, although she later admitted that she was hiding under the covers of her bed.

Stay strong, I texted her.

And then, slowly, the tension eased, and everything settled down. The hours passed, and nothing happened. Thursday had been a shit-storm at BMC. Reporters, family members, and celebrities were everywhere. Word went around that Oprah was going to be in the building the next day, that she wanted to meet with survivors. Mom came out of her shell at that one. Mom loves Oprah.

But even Oprah couldn't defy the lockdown, and on Friday the hospital was quiet. Without Mom, my aunts, and my dad, the atmosphere was peaceful, and I found myself drifting in and out of sleep. I still hated being alone, but maybe the nurses had been right all along; maybe I did need more time to rest.

Or maybe the way Tamerlan Tsarnaev died eased my mind.

My biggest fear had never been that we wouldn't catch the bombers. I had complete faith in the police. That's why I don't think my information was that important. Those guys were never going to get away with this. You don't bomb a marathon and walk away. Not in this city. The best I can say is that my information may have sped up the process.

My biggest fear was that the bombers would deny it. If Tamerlan Tsarnaev surrendered peacefully and proclaimed his innocence, it would have been a circus. I'd be in the news. I'd have to spend a year, at least, meeting with the FBI and being grilled by defense attorneys. I'd have to testify at his trial. Did I see this man at the site of the bombing? Yes. Did I see him with the backpack? Yes. Did I see the backpack explode? No, I didn't.

I know the FBI had pieces of the backpack that proved it contained the bomb. I know the bomb was remote-detonated by the control panel of a remote control car, so it would have been impossible to see both the bomb and the detonation device. But that small piece bothered me. How could I know for sure this guy was the killer, and not someone lucky enough to walk away at exactly the right time?

Tamerlan had settled that problem for me. When he executed MIT police officer Sean Collier, he revealed himself as a killer. A cold-blooded bastard. A man who was all business. He was willing to die for whatever he thought he was doing, whatever purpose he thought he was serving, and he did.

I slept easier on Friday, but not because Tamerlan Tsarnaev got what he deserved. I don't believe in retribution. I slept easier because he proved who he was.

I was still sleeping, off and on, when Kevin called around 3:00. The shelter-in-place order had been extended to the whole city, and nobody had been out of the hospital all day. So Kevin smuggled my relatives down an alley to a sushi restaurant that had agreed to open just for them and treated them to a gorgeous meal.

On the way back, the five of them stopped in the middle of Washington Street, one of the busiest roads in Boston, and took a photo. It was 4:00 on a Friday afternoon. There wasn't a single person around.

Thank you Kevin, I texted him, after Uncle Bob's kids told me what he had done.

You're welcome, he replied. And thank you for calling me Kevin.

———————

Erin arrived around 4:30. She had left her apartment before the lifting of the curfew, with the permission of the FBI. It was a five-mile drive, and she hadn't seen more than four or five people on the roads.

Like me, she seemed energized by the day—not to mention her first good shower in a week. She had pulled herself together and, despite the tension of the manhunt, used the forced break to organize my affairs.

She had asked her friend Kat, who worked in public relations, to handle our media requests. We weren't paying her, and she had never even met me, but Kat agreed immediately.

Aunt Jenn was designated my liaison to the "Jeff Bauman" Facebook page started by the couple I didn't know in Colorado. The page had a hundred thousand friends, so it had become the main source for updates and donations. So many people had been following my story, in fact, that other strangers were now posting links and photographs. Aunt Jenn wanted to help me, and she wanted to make sure I wasn't taken advantage of, so monitoring the page was a perfect task for her.

Uncle Bob talked to his lawyer friends about setting up an official charity and handling the money. When I was well enough, the lawyers would establish a trust in my name. Until then, the money would be held in a monitored bank account.

Now Erin had only one final thing to worry about: me. The second suspect hadn't been caught yet, but there were rumors on social media of shots fired (later proved untrue). We sat on my bed and watched the coverage together until, just before 10:00, it was announced that the second suspect had been captured alive.

You could hear the cheer, even in my fifth-floor hospital room. As soon as the news broke, people started pouring out of their houses toward public places, overjoyed to have their city back. Erin and I watched it live on television: a quiet vigil on Boylston Street, raucous Northeastern University students waving flags and hugging police officers. Boston Common filled up with people cheering and clapping. In Dorchester, where Martin Richard had lived, they were setting off fireworks.

"It's over," Erin said. She paused. "At least this part."

I put my arm around her. My upper body had healed enough by then, just barely, for us to lean on each other.

"Don't worry, E," I told her, as they showed the church bells ringing in Watertown. "Our kids will have legs."

10.

The next day, the Red Sox returned to Boston for the first time since the bombing. It was an afternoon game, on a perfect sunny Saturday. The crowds arrived early for a pregame ceremony in honor of victims and first responders. The phrase Boston Strong, seen throughout the city, had a new variation. You could see it on shirts and signs throughout Fenway: We Are Boston Strong. But it wasn't until they handed the microphone to David "Big Papi" Ortiz, the Red Sox's biggest star for the last ten years, that the meaning of that phrase was hammered home. It's known as The Speech, but it was only a few lines, made up on the spot:

> This jersey that we wear today, it doesn't say "Red Sox." It says "Boston." We want to thank you, Mayor Menino, Governor Patrick, the whole police department, for the great job that they did this past week. This is our fucking city! And nobody's going to dictate our freedom. Stay strong.

Our city. Our freedom. We are Boston, together, and we are strong. It was the perfect end to a terrible week, people said, but I didn't see The Speech, at least not live. I've seen it numerous times on the Internet since, but when David Ortiz actually spoke those words, I was with a physical therapist, learning how to put on my underpants.

Roll to one side, she taught me. Then back to the other. Then back again.

Life skills. That's what they called it. I was transferring to the secondary ICU, so I needed life skills. As the Red Sox fell behind the Kansas

City Royals, I was practicing pulling myself up with the help of my bed rack and sliding my underwear the last few inches up to my waist.

As they rallied with a home run in the eighth, I was working on getting out of bed. This involved a special tool: a wooden board. And not a special board, either, but a sanded and finished plank. I'd place it between the edge of the bed and the arm of a chair, then scoot into position and press down on it with my arms. This created enough force to lift my body and "transfer" it into the chair.

It was tough, trusting my arms like that. If I fell, there was nothing to catch me. I'd go straight to the floor, hips first if I was lucky, face-first if I wasn't. It happened. Of course, it happened. When you push yourself, sometimes you fall. And the pain was excruciating. Hitting my legs on the ground was like hitting open nerves with a sledgehammer.

"It feels great," I said, when I transferred into the chair for the first time. "I'm ready for more."

Ten minutes later, I was flat on my back in bed. The pain was so intense, I didn't feel like I ever wanted to get up again.

"That's normal," the specialist told me. "Your legs are so damaged, it will hurt to sit for a while."

"How long is a while?"

"Maybe a month."

No way. I wasn't waiting a month. I practiced my transfers, and I practiced, until the board chipped, and I got a splinter in my ass. (Nope, I wasn't wearing my underpants.) Talk about the difficulties of new technology! Fortunately, the hospital had another board.

By Sunday, I was already thinking of the next step: going to the bathroom. I was tired of crapping in a bedpan and peeing in a tube. So they brought a little portable toilet for beside the bed.

I used it once.

If I can do that, I thought, I can sit on a real toilet.

If I can sit on a toilet, I thought, after my first successful visit, I can get into a wheelchair.

That evening, my dad and stepmom brought me a gift: baggy workout shorts and a workout shirt. Easy clothes to put on for a guy with no legs.

"We thought this might help," Big Csilla said.

"Oh yeah," I said, almost snatching them out of her hand. Why hadn't I thought of this before?

By Monday, I was feeling frisky. "Let's go for a ride," I said to Chris and Tim, who had stayed with me the previous night.

We snuck in a wheelchair. I don't know if it was sneaking, really. We just didn't check with the nurses. I put my board down between the bed and the chair and hoisted myself in. A clean transfer, no problem.

I wheeled myself out of the room, waving to the nurses at their station. I'm back in the world, I thought.

I had never seen the hallway. It was much quieter than I expected. The fever had broken, I suppose, and the press had moved on. I saw Big D in the visitors' lounge, but he didn't see me, so I rolled slowly past him without saying a word. When he noticed me, his mouth hit the floor.

Kevin, who was with him in the visitors' lounge, started crying.

"How do you feel?" he asked.

"I feel like I can fly."

It was exactly two minutes past one week since the bombing, according to Kevin, which sounds like something he would notice. He and Big D had been discussing my future (I imagine Kevin was doing most of the talking), and when they saw me in my wheelchair, and I looked so happy, with this big smile on my face, Kevin lost it. He compared it to seeing your child walk for the first time.

Kevin's gay, in a long-term relationship, with no plans to adopt. Sometimes, it almost feels like he has adopted me.

We chatted for a while, Big D and I mostly taking the piss out of Kevin for being so emotional. That had always been our way in big moments, to defuse them with humor. But we were both pretty emotional, too.

Fortunately, a man interrupted us. He wanted to shake my hand. "I was there," he said. "I saw you lying on the ground." He paused. "I can't believe I'm talking to you now."

He had left out a sentence, but I knew what he meant: *I thought you were dead for sure.*

The man's name was Kevin Corcoran. He had been standing next to me, with his wife and daughter, when the first bomb went off. His wife, Celeste, had lost both her legs, the only other double amputee. She was really down about it, he admitted. She hated thinking about what her life would be like now. She had loved to walk on the beach. She had always been in charge. She hated feeling helpless. Their daughter, Sydney, was in the hospital bed next to her, but Celeste couldn't hold her. She couldn't tell her own daughter that everything was going to be okay. Sydney had almost bled to death on Boylston Street, but Kevin hadn't known it at the time. He couldn't find her in the chaos. He thought Sydney was okay, so he stayed with his wife. He knelt over her, hugging her. He thought she was going to die. She was covered with blood, and her feet were barely attached. Then they told him Sydney almost died, and that she might lose a leg, too. She was only seventeen.

"It helps to see you so happy, Jeff," he said, fighting back tears.

He shook my hand and walked back to his family's hospital room. I looked at Big D and Kevin. Then I turned and rolled down the hall, as far as I could, until I came to the window at the far end. Kevin caught up to me there.

"I'm proud of you," he said, putting his arm on my shoulder, like a father might after a difficult baseball game.

I was bawling. I was crying so hard that tears were streaming down my face. It was embarrassing.

"Look what they did," I said.

"It's okay to cry."

I couldn't have stopped, even if I'd wanted to. Outside, it was a beautiful day. I could see a garden, and downtown Boston in the distance. I could imagine the Red Sox out there at Fenway, and Ortiz calling Boston our fucking city.

"I'm not worried about me," I said. "I'm worried about the others. The ones who were hurt." I don't know if that's true. I think I was crying about everything. But I was thinking about Sydney Corcoran.

Kevin didn't say anything. He just let me cry.

"Why?" I said finally. "Why did they do this to us?"

RECOVERY

———•◆•———

11.

It was only after I moved to the secondary ICU that those kinds of thoughts started creeping in: Why? Why did this happen?

Why us?

And, more important, what could I have done?

That's the hardest part, looking at all the small decisions. What if we'd crossed the street to be with Erin's sister Jill? What if we hadn't walked down an extra block? Remy had moved toward the finish line only minutes before. What if Michele and I had joined her like she wanted us to? I had been about to suggest that to Michele when the bomb went off. What if the bomb had gone off one minute later? Would we all be fine now?

Or would things have been worse?

I think about the bomb all the time. How it blasted backward, away from the race. How because the bag was on the ground, the shrapnel came out low. My lower legs took a direct hit. They were so close to the bomb that they absorbed a huge amount of shrapnel. It instantly destroyed them—literally pulping my muscles and flesh—but that shielded people behind me. If my legs hadn't been in the way, more people might have died.

We were lucky. That's what the experts say about the death toll at the bombing. It could have been worse.

What if the shrapnel had come out higher? I was knocked out for a second after the blast. A few inches higher, and I never would have woken up.

What if I'd taken a step back? Would the shrapnel have destroyed my hips? That was what happened to Krystle Campbell. She was standing a few feet from me, just watching a race, but the shrapnel caught her higher, near the waist, and she died at the scene.

Or what if I'd gone to join Remy? What if I'd moved, and my legs hadn't been there, and another person had been killed? Or two? Or ten?

All of us have those thoughts. I know, because I've talked with other survivors. We all have questions. Why would God allow this to happen? Why would someone do this? I understand that this could happen, but how could it happen to me?

The harder question is: What if? What if I'd done something different? It's hard, because that feels like the question you can control.

It's not just the survivors. After the first week, when we finally had a chance to think, the doubts and guilt started to set in for all of us. My brother Chris thought he should have pushed for time off. My friend Sully said he should have been there, too. Remy was having nightmares, because she'd left Michele and me behind.

I still remember Erin saying that first time, "I'm sorry, Jeff. This is my fault."

"No," I said.

"If it hadn't been for me, you wouldn't have been there. I pushed you to go. I told you to meet me at the finish line. If it wasn't for me, you'd still have your legs."

"No, Erin, don't ever say that. It was my choice. I wanted to be there. I was proud to be there for you."

"But what if I hadn't run in the marathon? What if I hadn't slowed down? I should have been finished..."

"Erin, you didn't do anything wrong."

If anybody did something wrong, it was me.

I knew that guy was trouble. I knew he shouldn't have been there. What if I had...tackled him or something. You get those fantasies sometimes: *I stopped the bombing!* But of course that would never happen, tackling a stranger in a crowd.

What if I'd gone to the police? It was the finish line of the Boston Marathon; there were police officers everywhere.

But I wouldn't have had time. It happened too fast.

But I could have said something to him. That's the thought that haunted me. Tamerlan Tsarnaev looked right at me. He did that asshole thing, that stare where it's like, *Yeah, son, I'm in your space, what you gonna do about it?* Challenging me.

What if I'd said something to him? Not pick a fight, but just like "What's up?" What if I'd paid more attention? Made him feel uncomfortable? Would he have left the bomb if he thought I was watching him?

I know there's no point to this line of thought. Sure, it would have been great if I'd put the pieces together and acted. I'd have been a real hero. But that's not the way life works.

None of this was my fault. It was Tamerlan Tsarnaev's fault. He did this to us. Not God. Not random chance. Tamerlan. But what if...

Erin ate herself up for weeks, worrying about it. No matter how many times I said, "Never think that way, Erin. Never," she couldn't stop feeling guilty.

It's impossible not to. I mean, I'm not the type to dwell. What if my parents hadn't divorced? What if I'd finished college? I don't worry about those things. What's the point? I roll with what life gives me. I make the best of it.

But even I doubted during that second week. After the pain diminished, and especially after I started to meet other victims. Celeste and Sydney Corcoran were standing right beside me. So was John Odom, and Krystle Campbell, who had died. I didn't notice them at the time, but they were there, cheering for loved ones and strangers, having a great time. And now, if they were lucky, they were in the hospital, their lives blasted apart. Scared. Sad. Unsure of the future.

It wasn't just the story Mr. Corcoran told that affected me that day. It was the way he looked. He was so traumatized. There are some things you can never get over, and seeing your wife and daughter brutally injured seemed like one of them.

I don't cry for myself. I try not to be angry. I can deal with what happened, because it happened to me. But if the bombers had hurt Erin or Mom? If I was the one that had to look down at someone I loved in that hospital bed? That would be different. I would track those bastards into the grave.

I know Mr. Corcoran now, so I know I was wrong about him. He's not broken. He's Boston Strong. And he's proud. He has an amazing family. But in that hospital, that week, he looked as wounded as his wife.

I didn't do that to them. I never thought I did, and I never really blamed myself. But in those last minutes before the bomb went off, there was one person in the world who could have prevented all their pain. Only one. And that person was me.

Don't dwell on that, Jeff, I would tell myself. It's in the past. Focus on right now.

And I did. I may have lain awake at night, in pain and wondering about the future, but during the day, I was smiling.

12.

I was lucky. That's how I tried to look at it. I was standing right next to a bomb, and I survived.

I had health insurance. I had thousands of people who gave thousands of dollars to help me. I had top medical care—and, the doctors told me, one day I'd have the best artificial legs in the world, courtesy of a charitable fund.

I had an amazing girlfriend.

I had a giving family. Every day, Uncle Bob and Aunt Cathleen brought me home-cooked meals. Every other patient was eating Jell-O, while I was scarfing down beef chili and enchiladas.

"Where do you live, anyway?" I asked Kevin one morning when he brought my daily pastries. Anytime I needed something, I'd text Kevin, and he would be there in five minutes.

He went to the window, snapped a photo, and brought it back. "See that street?" he said. "That's my block." Kevin lived fourteen houses from the hospital.

Like I said, lucky.

By Tuesday of the second week, I could transfer into my wheelchair and roll around whenever I wanted. That was when I discovered that many victims hadn't yet been moved out of the emergency ICU. My injuries were so horrific that there wasn't any question about how to treat them. My legs had to come off. And since my knees couldn't be saved, the doctors cut diagonally through the thighs, allowing my leg wounds to seal properly.

Other people, who appeared less injured, went through multiple surgeries, trying to save their legs. Or they had severe burns, necessitating weeks in intensive care. Mr. Odom had eleven surgeries on his severed arteries. His wound was through his hip; otherwise, they would have amputated. The last victim to leave the hospital, Marc Fucarile, had metal lodged near his heart. He lost one leg and was under the knife sixteen times, for a total of forty-nine surgical procedures.

I also didn't have infections or complications, which can be as bad as the original injuries. My new friend Patrick, for instance, lost one leg below the knee. Having a knee is huge for amputees; it's more muscle, and it gives you control of another major joint. If you lose one leg below the knee, you'll be back to your normal life within weeks. Losing four joints, as I did, changes everything.

So it seemed like Patrick would have a much easier recovery than me. Except that in order to save his knee, doctors had to close his amputation with a skin graft.

The graft became infected, so he had another surgery to replace it. In fact, he had several more. Months later, he's having complications: the skin grafts keep ripping away when he uses his artificial leg. Imagine that you're walking along, and six inches of skin on your leg suddenly tears apart—and it keeps happening, again and again.

So I was lucky. Lucky that my wounds didn't become infected. Lucky that my surgery was straightforward and well performed.

Which isn't the same as saying it was easy. It wasn't. It straight up sucked. I hated looking at my thighs. Once, and only once, I lifted them with my hands to check out the bottoms of my legs. They were covered with blood and scabs. No wonder they hurt like hell.

In movies, a character takes a vicious beating, and the next day they stick an ice pack on a bruise and say they're sore. Five minutes later, they're chasing someone. But a week later, I still felt like my organs were pulped. That was what the doctors had worried about: that I was smashed inside. I guess I was lucky it only felt that way, even if I was still so messed up I couldn't even lie on my stomach. The foot-long slice where they opened me up was too raw.

That didn't keep me from the wheelchair, though. As soon as they moved me to my new room, I was rolling. I don't want to make too much of it. After all, I was just going up and down a hospital hallway. But I could visit people: not just the other victims, but their families, too.

And now that I was out of the emergency area, more people could visit me. A lot of my friends came by for the first time that week. My nephew Cole, who was seven, dropped in for a visit after school.

"Uncle Jeff," he said, with a serious-little-kid expression. "Are your legs going to grow back?"

"No they're not, Forehead," I said. That's what Derek and I call Cole: the Forehead. He's a cute kid, but he has a lot of real estate up there. "But don't worry. I'm going to get some bionic legs."

"Really?"

"Oh yeah. Don't mess with Uncle Jeff. I'm going to be a superhero."

Later, a huge African-American police officer came by. He wasn't built like Stevan Ridley, the New England Patriots running back, who had visited me the day after Julian Edelman did. Ridley was the most stacked guy I have ever seen.

"Do you work out every day?" I had asked him.

"Three times a day, buddy. Every day."

This officer was tall. He towered over me, especially since I was down in the chair. He had come to give me a few things that had been recovered at the scene. He could have sent them over, but I could tell he wanted to talk to me. He handed me a plastic bag. Inside were my driver's license and a credit card. They looked fine, not torn or burned or anything. I just sat there staring at them, not saying anything. It's weird, what survives.

"You okay, Jeff?" the officer asked.

"Yes, sir."

"Do you need anything?"

I looked at him sadly. "No, I'm all right."

"You sure?"

"It's just..."

"Name it, buddy."

I paused. "Do you think you can find my sneakers? I loved those sneakers."

The poor guy looked like he was about to faint. My sneakers had been destroyed, just like my feet. He didn't know what to say.

Until I laughed. "I'm just kidding," I said.

"Oh, man," he said. "You got me, Jeff. You really got me."

He was a nice guy. I feel like I keep saying that, but it's true. I met one bad person in this whole experience, but he's dead now. Everyone else was amazing: kind, caring, giving.

I'm coming out of this experience with damage. I guess you'd call it suspicion. I know how evil humans can be, and I'm watchful, because the bad dudes are out there.

But I know something else, too: bad people are rare.

Good people are everywhere.

13.

Wednesday, April 24, was Sydney Corcoran's eighteenth birthday. Erin had bought her a card, and when she came in that morning, she wanted me to sign it. I had never met Sydney, but I had heard her story from her father and others. She had been in a car accident at sixteen that cracked her skull. Now, a little more than a year later, she was dealing with a severe leg injury.

"A card?!" I said. "I've got to give her something more."

My room was filling up with flowers and gifts. My location hadn't been made public, and Aunt Jenn had only recently posted a P.O. box address on Facebook, so these were mostly from friends and coworkers: small electronics, headphones, a guitar from a close friend. The media buyers at the Costco corporate office in Seattle had sent me a care package, so my table was full of movies, magazines, and books.

And then there was my mandolin. My dad had mentioned my love of music in a newspaper article, so Guitar Center offered me a free guitar. But I was having trouble playing the two—one from a friend, one from home—that I already had. My damaged eardrums distorted the sound, and the echoes gave me a headache. I played at the hospital mostly to keep people from worrying. I didn't want them to know how difficult it was to do something I used to love.

So Guitar Center gave me a mandolin instead. I loved that mandolin; it sat beside my bed for weeks, in a place of honor. I couldn't imagine giving away any of my instruments, even to another bombing victim.

Besides, I didn't know if Sydney liked music.

Then I saw the tablet computer. Someone in senior management at

Costco had sent it to me a few days after the bombing. It was the first computer I had ever owned. On Monday, I had used it to FaceTime with my department manager, Maya, who was visiting family in Holland the week of the bombing.

It went so well that Kevin set up a FaceTime call with our Costco store. The regional vice president flew in to spend the morning with me, and they put us on the big-screen television in the break room.

Everyone came, even people who had the day off. Some even brought their children.

"We love you, Jeff!" a little boy said.

I was laughing. There was a big banner that looked like kindergarteners had made it (by the way, kindergarteners make awesome banners) and a cake with a guitar and the famous Boston "B" on it.

"We're doing this for you," they said as they stuffed their faces.

"Sure, Jeff, we get the cake. But you get the vacation."

"Vacation forever!" I said. I looked at Kevin, who was laughing. "I'm just kidding, guys. I'm coming back. Just not today."

I actually didn't know if I was going back. My old job involved a lot of walking and standing. There was no way I could do it anymore. But that wasn't my concern right then. I was just happy to see the old crew.

The tablet was the nicest thing I'd been given, so I wanted Sydney to have it. She deserved it more than me. But I changed my mind at the last second. The tablet had personal value, since it had been given by friends.

I chose some portable speakers instead. I stuck them in a gift bag, along with Erin's card, and rolled across the hall to Sydney's room. She was sitting up in a chair, with her heavily bandaged leg propped in front of her. There were two birthday balloons and a few relatives, but otherwise it was just a normal day at BMC. Sydney had already received the best birthday gift possible: the doctors had saved her leg.

I gave her my package. It was a bit of a stretch, because I couldn't get my wheelchair past her leg. Right as we both had our hands on it, someone snapped a picture. I hear you can see it on the Internet now. Of course you can. You can see everything on the Internet. But it was originally posted to the Celeste and Sydney Recovery Fund website, so I don't mind. If the photo helps with the Corcorans' medical bills, then it's more than I ever hoped to give.

That night, I received my own gift, when a Hispanic man with long, curly hair walked into my room. I would have known him immediately, even without his famous cowboy hat, because I could never forget his face. It was Carlos Arredondo, the man who saved my life.

Carlos was famous; he had been all over the news. There was another picture of him, holding a torn and bloody American flag in the moments after he rescued me, that was almost as famous in Boston as the iconic shot of us together.

"Carlos!" I yelled when I saw him in the doorway.

He smiled and came toward me, and I couldn't help myself, I reached out and hugged him. Carlos is a hugger. He's always smiling, always wanting to step close and talk. It hurt, but I didn't want to let him go. What can you say to the man who gave you everything? I said, "Thank you," but that wasn't enough.

He gave me a hat and a handwritten sign: Together Strong. He asked how I was doing. I showed him the scars and burns on my back. We discussed my goals and chatted about my recovery. I asked him about his life. At first he didn't want to talk about himself, but eventually, he told me his story.

Carlos was born in Costa Rica. He had come to this country illegally, but his two sons, Alex and Brian, were born in the Jamaica Plain section of Boston and were American citizens. His oldest son, Alex, entered the Marines at age seventeen, straight out of high school. He loved the Marines. He loved the idea of serving his country. The Marines were going to pay for him to go to college.

Three years later, a van pulled up to Carlos's house in Florida, where he had moved after a divorce. It was August 24, 2004, his forty-fourth birthday. He was expecting a birthday call from Alex. Instead, three Marines told him his son was dead. He had been killed by a sniper in Iraq.

Carlos told me he wasn't sure what happened next. He just went crazy with grief. He wanted to be alone, but the Marines wouldn't leave his front yard until his wife—Alex's stepmom—came home. He became agitated, then angry. He went into the garage, grabbed a gas can and a blowtorch, and locked himself in the front seat of the Marines' van. He doused himself with gasoline and set himself on fire. He denied it later, but I think he was trying to kill himself. Instead, the van exploded, hurling him onto his front lawn, on fire. The Marines saved his life. He was severely burned on 26 percent of his body, but he attended his son's funeral on a stretcher. He asked to be lifted onto the casket. He lay on top of it and apologized to Alex, because he had done nothing, he said, to save him.

He went through months of physical recovery and legal trouble. Some people wanted him prosecuted for destruction of government property. He was in agony from the burns. He didn't care. He thought only of his son and how he hadn't helped him.

"I let him die."

When he was well enough, he put a message on his pickup truck: "Alexander Arredondo. My Son. KIA in Iraq." He put American flags in the bed, along with his son's uniform and a photograph from his funeral. He quit his construction job and drove around the country, speaking out against the war.

He was beaten up. He was spit on and called racist names. He was told to go back to wherever he came from. He kept attending rallies, sometimes pulling a coffin draped in an American flag and his son's uniform, sometimes carrying Alex's desert boots and dog tags. He stood in front of the White House with a picture of Alex in his coffin, wearing his dress blues. He talked to anyone who would listen.

His younger son, Brian, was struggling with depression. The boys had been joined at the hip, Carlos told me. Brian idolized Alex. He took his death hard. Carlos moved back to the Boston area to be near Brian, who lived with his mother, and Alex's grave. In 2006, Carlos became a United States citizen. He legally changed his name to Alexander Brian Arredondo, in honor of his sons.

But the war dragged on, and Brian's depression grew worse. He fell into drugs and struggled with addiction. "He was tortured by his brother's death. That's what his mother always said. Brian was tortured."

On December 19, 2011, Brian Arredondo committed suicide. It was seven years since his brother died in Najaf, and only a few days before the last troops came home from Iraq.

By that time, I was crying. Carlos gave me a tissue, then reached into his pocket. "I live for them," he said.

He handed me his card. It read in part:

Carlos Arredondo
Dad on Fire

He had been at the finish line of the Boston Marathon handing out American flags. He was there to support the "Tough Ruck" team, twenty National Guardsmen who had started marching the marathon route with rucksacks at 5:30 a.m. They were raising money for the families of soldiers killed in action, or those who had committed suicide or died in PTSD-related accidents. One of the guardsmen was marching in honor of Alex.

The soldiers had just crossed the finish line, after nine hours of marching, when the first bomb went off. Carlos saw the ball of fire. He saw a man fall over the barricade into the marathon course. And then everything disappeared into smoke. He jumped the barricade on his side and was halfway across the road when the second bomb exploded.

He crossed himself, *God protect me*, and kept running. He was lifting the barricade off Michele when he saw me, without my legs, lying in a pool of blood. He knew I didn't have much time. He lifted me into the wheelchair. He ran beside me, unwilling to leave my side. He stayed with me as long as he could, staring after the ambulance as it pulled away and headed down the street. I was the one person he focused on that day.

By then, we were both crying. I hugged him again, and he hugged me back. There was a long silence, the only time I've been around Carlos when he wasn't talking.

"Don't cry," he said, wiping away his tears. "Something good happened."

English is Carlos's second language, so it's sometimes hard for him to express the nuances. What he said probably sounds strange to you. But in context, I knew exactly what he meant. He meant that something good had happened *because he was alive.* I suspect it had been hard for him since Alex's death. He believed he was doing the right thing, but it was probably hard to know if it was making a difference. The war never ended. He lost his other son.

But he saved my life. I mean that: I would be dead today without Carlos Arredondo. And now he can say to himself, if he ever struggled with it before: Something good happened because of me. It's a good thing I survived.

14.

I transferred from Boston Medical to the Spaulding Rehabilitation Center the day after I met Carlos. Erin had pulled strings to get me transferred quickly, because she thought it would lift my spirits. And she was right. It felt like a big deal to leave the hospital, even if I was still, technically, in a hospital. It was a vote of confidence from my doctors. My treatment wouldn't be about my immediate health anymore; it would be about learning how to live without legs.

I was all in on that, because I was already sick of the wheelchair. I wanted to walk.

At first, they transferred me to the old Spaulding Rehab Center, a plain redbrick building squeezed between the TD North office tower and the Zakim Bridge on the northwest edge of downtown. It was cramped and worn down and felt like an old mental hospital, complete with metal gates that could be pulled down at the ends of the hall. I felt like I'd been rolled into *The Shining*.

Even the television sucked. It was an old tube TV, not a flat-screen, and the picture was so bad the Red Sox looked green.

Three days later, they strapped me and a few other patients into a special van and drove us a mile or two north, through an old neighborhood, then through an industrial area, then finally onto a long block of new buildings. The new Spaulding Rehabilitation Center was on the site of the old navy yard, on the point of land where the Mystic River met the bay. It was a world-class facility, in planning and construction for ten years, and it happened to open twelve days after the bombing.

They took us through the front door, where backhoes were leveling the land for a park next door. The floors gleamed, and the hallways were extrawide, so two wheelchairs could pass with ease. My room on the fifth floor had a view across the river to the old docks and warehouses on the north side, and the windows were low enough that I could look out of them from my wheelchair. This was progress. I couldn't see well out of the medical center windows, and at the old Spaulding . . . forget it. I heard they'd originally designed the windows at "standing person" height at the new Spaulding, too, meaning you couldn't look directly out the window if you were sitting down. Your line of sight was too low. A guy in a wheelchair pointed out the problem. It cost $300,000 to lower the windowsills.

Best of all, each patient room had a bathroom, and I could roll to the sink and into the shower with ease. The bathrooms at Boston Medical were supposedly wheelchair friendly, but they were small. It was like being in an airplane bathroom. I was always banging into things, feeling trapped, and forgetting which little compartment served what purpose. New Spaulding was like going from a Boeing 747 to the USS *Enterprise*.

The building was better for my family, too. Much better. There was a nice visitors' lounge at the end of my hall, with views of the river. There was a decent cafeteria on the first floor, and space in my room for five or six guests. That night, Erin slept on the sofa at the foot of my bed, the first time in two weeks she was able to stretch out. Not that she got a good night's sleep. I was still in pain whenever I rolled over, and more than once Erin climbed into bed and comforted me, talking and rubbing my singed afro hair.

The next day, Erin's roommate, Michele, moved into the room next to mine. As I was being evacuated from the bombing site, Michele had been rushed to the marathon medical tent. Shrapnel had shredded the lower part of her right leg. The EMT didn't think they could save it. At Beth Israel Deaconess Medical Center, they planned to amputate her foot. Two emergency surgeries saved her leg and foot, but her Achilles tendon was so damaged she couldn't walk. The first time she tried, on

Thursday, she managed only two steps. Erin had been back and forth all week to see her at Beth Israel Deaconess, including for her skin-graft surgery on Friday.

Having both of us at Spaulding made things easier for Erin. Her life, or at least this part of it, was finally manageable. She could be there for both her best friend and her boyfriend without driving across town.

It made it easier on Michele and me, too. We hadn't seen each other since locking eyes after the bombing; I was so happy she was alive. She felt the same about me, considering she'd seen me lying in a pool of blood. Early in the morning, when neither of us could sleep, we'd sit together and talk about what had happened. I told her about seeing bone through the hole in her leg. She told me about realizing my legs were gone.

"I had a bad feeling about the guy," I told her. "I was about to say we should move." She hadn't known that. It made me feel guilty again.

"I still smell it," I told her one morning. "People were on fire."

"I know," she said. And she did. Only someone who was there could understand the horror of the smell. That was what was great about having Michele next door.

In the afternoon, we'd usually hang out with Erin. Sometimes we'd watch television. Sometimes I'd play my mandolin. Or I'd do wheelies, which always impress girls. We talked more than we ever had before. Michele is a talker, and I am quiet by nature. I don't think she really knew me until we sat with Erin in her room.

Late in the week, Remy came for a visit. She had an ugly shrapnel wound in her thigh, and the doctors had surgically implanted a valve in her leg to drain the pus. She had spent time at Spaulding, but was now home with her parents in Amesbury.

Remy had deeply conflicted feelings. Because of her wound, she was often in pain. Like the rest of us, she had trouble sleeping. And she felt guilty about leaving Michele and me behind when she went toward the finish line. She felt she should have been there with us, although if she had been, nothing would have been better. It would have just been three of us severely injured, instead of two.

Her father had been quoted in the newspaper a few days after the bombing saying she was "angry and depressed." It was no doubt true. We all felt angry and depressed. Sometimes one, sometimes the other, sometimes both. But now Remy was conflicted about that, too.

"I'm embarrassed," she confided to Erin. "Why should I be struggling when other people have it so much worse?"

Knowing Remy, she's probably embarrassed that I'm writing about this. But she shouldn't be, because her feelings are normal. That's what I've come to realize. Feeling guilty—whether about being lucky or about not stopping the bomber—is normal. So is embarrassment. I still feel embarrassed every day because I don't have legs. So is feeling traumatized. Being twenty feet from a bomb instead of two doesn't make it easy.

We didn't talk about that, though. There was no need. We talked about our lives. Our recoveries. Our families.

"Are you part of the family?" a nurse had asked Michele's boyfriend when she found them together in her room on the second day.

"No," he said. "This is our fifth date."

"It wasn't easy having my boyfriend put me on the bedside commode for our fifth date," Michele told us with a laugh.

Before the bombing, she hadn't been using the word *boyfriend*. Now, she relied on him. Like Erin and me, they were closer because of what they'd been through. I don't know if that's a natural reaction to tragedy: to move toward someone, if they don't pull away.

I tend to think tragedy gives you perspective. When I was lying in my emergency room bed with no legs, staring at the ceiling, I had to ask myself: What do I want now? What do I care about?

When I am in pain, who makes me feel better? Who can I be honest with, without being afraid of their reaction? The answer always came up Erin.

I felt better when she was there, so much so that the only photograph in my hospital room was of her. It was a cell phone shot I'd taken in Washington, D.C., a close-up of the two of us pressed together and smiling. I taped it to my IV stand so I would see it every time I opened my eyes.

That day with Michele and Remy was important, especially for Erin. With the four of us together, I think she felt her own wound healing. Damage had been done, but the essential parts of her life had not been lost. She still had her family and friends. She still had her handsome man. The world she had made for herself had been blown off center, sure, but she was stronger because of what we'd been through.

Someone snapped a picture of the four of us that day. There are at least a dozen pictures of the four of us together, spread out over the last year and a half, but that picture is my favorite. Michele's in bed with her leg in a walking boot. Remy is standing to one side of her, and Erin is sitting on the bed on her other side. I'm beside Erin, in my wheelchair, with my mandolin, ready to play.

And we're smiling. Not photograph smiles, but genuine smiles, like we're about to start laughing. It looks like we're having a good time.

Unbreakable. That was the word Michele's father used. He told her, "I feel like, because of what we've been through, our family is unbreakable."

I think it was the same for the four of us. I hope we always stay that way.

15.

Spaulding was . . . I want to say it was a community, because that was where the bombing victims came together. We had been spread out at the five hospitals near downtown Boston, but most of us eventually ended up at Spaulding. Not all of us, of course. I only saw the daughter from the Richard family once, for instance, even though she lost a leg. That family had suffered like nobody else: the mother had eye damage, the little girl lost her leg, and poor Martin Richard, who was eight years old, was killed. I saw his older brother once, and it broke my heart. He was the saddest kid I have ever met.

Mom cries every time she thinks of them. "They watched their son die," she says.

"Martin was Boston Strong," the family said in their lone statement to the press. That's the only time those words choked me up. And they've never made me more proud.

But Spaulding wasn't a community. It was the Island of Misfit Toys. Nobody wanted to be there, but we were broken, so we had nowhere else to go. Spaulding was not a jolly place, even though they tried to make it as jolly as they could.

And just like the toys on the island, we all had one goal: to get out.

I started working on that the first day. I had been practicing my transfers at Boston Medical, so by the time I reached Spaulding I no longer needed my board. I could easily slide from my bed to my wheelchair, then onto my mat in the gym, which was more like a single bed covered in a sheet than those mats you nap on in kindergarten.

I still couldn't lie on my stomach because of my surgical wound, so my therapist, Carlyn Wells, told me to lie on my side. She grabbed my leg and pulled it backward as far as she could. At first I almost screamed. It hurt for her to touch my leg, much less pull on it, but once I got over the shock it felt so good. My muscles had tightened up from two weeks of lying in bed, but also from the shock of the blast. It was like my body had clenched, then never let go. It felt so good for Carlyn to pull me apart.

After the stretch, while I was still lying on my side, she asked me to lift my right leg. Higher, she said. Higher. I could lift it only a few times.

I rolled over on my other side and lifted my left leg. It was even weaker than the right.

I sat up and I worked on leg lifts from a seated position. I hated looking at my legs. They were like dancing sausages, with bandages over the ends. Ten lifts, and I was sweating.

"It's not weakness, it's muscle trauma," Carlyn told me. "Although you do need to get stronger."

I lifted free weights with my arms: curls, shoulder shrugs, extensions.

"Everything is connected," Carlyn told me.

I hadn't just lost my legs; I'd changed the role of each muscle in my body. Sitting up was harder without legs, because I had to rely on my core. Balance meant squaring and lifting my shoulders, not just setting my thighs. When you walk, you can slump your upper body, because your leg muscles can compensate. It's not a good way to walk, but most people do it that way, at least some of the time. I wasn't going to be able to "take steps off" anymore. I had to be upright and strong, because my new legs would be more like stilts than the bionics I had promised my nephew Cole. They would support me, but only my upper body would keep them beneath me.

Since I couldn't sleep, I chose the first training session of the morning. It was about two hours long, so I was usually done by 10:30. Soon after, when I was most tired, a speech therapist would come to my room. Mostly, we talked. At the end, she gave me five words, then came back an hour later and asked me what they were. When that wasn't a problem, she gave me ten more, then came back the next day and asked me to repeat them. She gave me math homework.

"Why are you doing this?" I asked her. "Your job is stupid." I was joking with her, but only partially. I knew she was testing for brain damage, and I hated it.

"You're fine," she told me after a week of torture.

Then there was psychological counseling, both individual and group. And occupational therapy designed to help me find solutions for practical chores.

Mom and Aunt Jenn always arrived in the late morning. (My dad had the evening shift, and it was better if they never saw each other.) Mom had taken time off from work to be with me, but there wasn't much she could do. She fidgeted around the room, asking me questions, but I was often frustrated, and I didn't feel like talking.

Fortunately, there was the mail. Aunt Jenn had put her address on the Facebook page, and cards and gifts had come flooding in. She packed them up every morning, then picked up Mom and drove her to Spaulding. Mom didn't like driving in the city.

I couldn't believe the nice things people wrote. Or how much they cared. Most of them weren't even from Boston, but they had been following my story, and they wanted to help. Businesses were donating a portion of their sales; small towns were holding fund-raisers; families were pooling resources. Letters would include checks for hundreds of dollars.

A hundred dollars, for a stranger? That's a big deal.

"How can that be, Mom?" I asked.

"Jeffrey," Mom said, holding my hand as if she was delivering bad news, "people have given you more than $100,000."

A hundred thousand dollars?! I had dropped out of college over a $900 debt. I had been making less than $16,000 a year. Now people had donated $100,000 to help me, just because my legs had been pulverized?

It's stupid to say I would have traded the money for my legs. Of course I would have. But I wasn't even thinking like that. I was too overwhelmed.

And it's stupid to focus just on the money.

A woman living in Japan sent me a tiny replica of samurai armor. How cool is that?

A man from Bend, Oregon, sent me a custom Epiphone Les Paul Gibson guitar. It was olive colored and stripped down, the most beautiful guitar I had ever seen, but the note made it one of a kind:

> I read about what happened to you and what you are going through, and although you don't know me, I wanted you to know I'm thinking about you and sending prayers your way.... I read that you like to play guitar, so I'm sending you one that has been special to me. It's nothing fancy, but it has a great tone and a good action on it. After a while, I have found that guitars become like old friends—consider this a gift from a new one....

It wasn't just adults who gave from the heart. A ten-year-old boy broke open his piggy bank and sent me all his money. It was almost $20 in small bills and change.

"Send him a PlayStation," I said.

"You can't do that, Jeff," Mom said.

"Why not?"

"You can't buy something for everyone that gives to you."

"Why not?"

Mom picked up another letter and read it: "'I'm sure you've heard this over and over again by now, but you are truly a hero. I just want to thank you for being an inspiration to this entire nation. I've never seen a stronger, more resilient person in my life.'"

"I don't understand," I said. "Why do people say that about me?"

Mom looked at me. I hated being looked at. Did all those people writing letters know that? If they did, what would they have thought?

"They admire your bravery," Mom said.

I wanted to say, *But I'm not brave. I just lost my legs.*

I mean, some kid, in some other state, saved his money for years, probably taking the dishes off the table and putting his clean clothes away, doing chores for his mom. He saved up, probably to buy one of those *Despicable Me* minions or something—kids love the minions, right? I have a minion sticker on my wheelchair. Cole gave it to me.

But does the kid buy the minion? No.

He gives his money to a stranger.

And it wasn't only that kid. There were dozens of kids who sent me their allowance money. Kindergarten classes drew me pictures. Kids sold their toys to raise funds for bombing victims. "This is so you can feel better," they wrote.

Maybe someday I'll start a charity. I'll find kids who have done something kind, and I'll give them a gift in return, because that's real bravery, caring so much about someone else.

No, I guess that's stupid. There are better ways to show that kindness matters. And it does. Nothing makes you happier than a kid writing to say you are their hero.

But it was also hard. People would write and tell me, "You are Boston Strong, Jeff." Or "You are what makes this country great." Or "I know if you can make it through this, Jeff, that means we'll all be okay."

But what if I didn't make it? What if I broke down?

What if people saw how frustrated the little things made me?

The workouts were punishing. By the time I had advanced to thigh lifts, my legs were burning. I had to lie on my side and lift each leg ten times, but there were days I couldn't do it. My muscles weren't ready. They would clench and spasm. I had to pound on my legs, digging my thumbs into my thighs to loosen the muscles, or the pain would keep getting worse.

At times like that, I wondered, What if I quit?

What if I just accepted the chair?

What if I never felt normal again?

I was never a subscriber to the "no pain, no gain" school of life. Doctors had to confiscate weights from one guy in Spaulding, who was injured in a snowmobile accident, so he wouldn't work out unsupervised in his room. He kept asking and asking, so they let him be the first patient to enter the new building. He was wearing an American flag shirt when he rolled through the door.

What if the world expected me to be that guy?

It wasn't my personality. I was never competitive. I was just... ordinary. I played softball in a league, but mostly for the beer. I loved pickup basketball games, but I didn't particularly care if we won.

Baseball was my game, even if I wasn't the best player. That was my cousin, Big D. Derek got a full ride to Bridgeport University in Connecticut, where he was a four-year starter. He was a big left-handed pitcher. He didn't strike out a lot of guys, maybe because his fastball was only in the high eighties, but he'd knock them down, inning after inning. I thought he was going pro for sure, but he never got the call. That was how he ended up paving roads for Uncle Bob.

My half brothers on my dad's side, Chris and Alan, were hockey players. My dad even built a hockey rink in the backyard. He used marine-grade plywood for the walls at each end and a wooden frame to hold the ice, and every year around Thanksgiving, when I was up for a visit and it was freezing in Concord, he'd say, "Let's go set it up, boys."

We'd work the whole weekend nailing supports into the boards, while Dad flooded the frame, let the water harden into ice, then flooded it again. He'd do that maybe fifteen times, so the ice would stay solid all winter. It was usually about midnight when he finally turned on the big floodlights, connected by extension cords to the house, and lit up our work. Chris could stay out there all night in short sleeves, even though it was minus twenty degrees. He had a ninety-mile-an-hour slapshot, and he'd work on it for hours. I think if he hadn't gotten off track, he could have played for a Division I college.

I usually lasted twenty minutes. Then the chill got to me, and I had to call it a night.

But that wasn't an option now. No matter how much it hurt, there was no way I could settle for the chair.

Maybe it would have been different if I'd been in a car accident. Then I wouldn't have had so many people watching me, and hoping for me, and caring about whether I succeeded.

Then my injuries wouldn't have been intentional. They wouldn't have been the work of people who were trying to hurt me and destroy my life. People I could never let win.

Maybe if it had been an accident, I would have given in to the fear, because knowing your life is different, and that a huge part of you is missing forever...that's terrifying. Alone at night, I'd sometimes think, Screw it, Jeff. It's too much. How can they expect you to keep getting up from this?

It's easier, after all, to lie down and accept your fate, especially when your legs are throbbing and your burns are rubbed raw.

But I'd think of all the people out there, rooting for me. I'd think of the kids, kneeling beside their beds, saying prayers for my recovery. And the next day, I'd be back on the arm bicycle, pedaling faster, or I'd be pushing myself to do ten leg lifts this time, then eleven, then twelve.

You can do it, Jeff. It's not just about you. It's not just for you.

You're Boston Strong.

16.

Before Spaulding, I tried to stay out of the media. During my second week at BMC, Kat gave me a list of one hundred interview requests and asked if I wanted to do any of them. I chose one: *GQ* magazine, which was putting together an article about the effort to save lives that included six main points of view. Why did I choose *GQ*? I don't know. I've never read the magazine. But it's a *gentleman's* quarterly, right? That sounds classy to me.

That article wouldn't come out for more than a month, though, so my first public comments happened at old Spaulding, when I did an interview with Gerry Callahan for local sports radio station WEEI. I didn't think about it too much. Mr. Callahan had grown up in Chelmsford, and he was my uncle Bob's lifelong best friend. I had known him since I was a little kid, and I still remember when he came to my third-grade class to talk to us.

If you listen to his show, you probably know about his character Bob the Drunk. That's my uncle! "Highly fictionalized," Uncle Bob insists, "highly fictionalized"—but I don't know if I believe him.

So why wouldn't I talk with Mr. Callahan? It was only a five-minute phone interview, and I could do it from my hospital bed. The conversation got a little deep at times, especially for a cutup like Gerry Callahan, but it was fun. Mostly, we just chatted about how I was doing.

Well, people blew up. A few liberals didn't like it, I guess, because Gerry Callahan is conservative, and they made a bit of a stink about politicizing things, or something like that, I don't know.

Mostly, though, it was other media. They couldn't believe I had turned down network news, Oprah Winfrey, and the *Boston Globe* to give an exclusive to local sports radio. But it wasn't an exclusive, and it wasn't a political statement. It was just a favor for Uncle Bob.

"Ah, just let it go," I said, when reporters started pressing for an explanation. "I don't feel like dealing with it." I guess I was naive. I didn't think anyone would care what I said. Now that I realized people were probably going to overreact, I figured it was best to keep quiet.

Besides, I'd already agreed to one other feature interview, and it wasn't with the *Boston Globe*, even though they were the biggest newspaper in town and, in some ways, this was our story together. A lot of reporters, from all kinds of media sources, were aggressive or disrespectful of our privacy, especially in that first week. Erin's sister Gail caught an ABC reporter in Boston Medical Center eavesdropping on family conversations and trying to strike up casual conversations. Another reporter tried to enter a survivor's therapy session that Remy was attending. Early Friday morning, during the manhunt, a reporter called Erin's mom and, as a pressure tactic, implied that talking with him would be helpful to finding the missing suspect.

Kat had a run-in with a *Boston Globe* reporter who was working on a big article centered on a time line of the first week. We had asked Kat not to give any information to the media, so she told the reporter she couldn't comment on my role in identifying the bombers. He responded that if she wouldn't comment, then he could question the Facebook page that was my main source of donations. There were dozens of ways to give to victims that first week, and some were sketchy at best. Kat knew that any doubt expressed by a leading newspaper could affect the site, but she held firm, just as we'd asked.

The reporter for the *New York Times*, Tim Rohan, was different. My brother Chris had met him outside Boston Medical, and he had written a nice article about my dad. Dad brought Tim to my room the next day, and we chatted. Tim didn't ask for an interview or try to sell himself to me. Mostly, we talked about the Red Sox, who were off to a surprising hot start and in first place. Like me, Tim was a big baseball fan.

He was also a twenty-three-year-old intern.

Before the bombing, the *New York Times*, apparently, hadn't thought much of the Boston Marathon. It was a great event, but a boring story. The same every year. So they sent one intern from their sports department to cover it. Tim Rohan was the only *New York Times* reporter on the scene for one of the biggest events of the year.

And to the paper's credit, they let him run with it. They didn't send a big shot for follow-up interviews. They let Tim handle it the way he wanted to. And it worked, at least with me.

When Kat suggested I agree to one big article to tell my story, I instantly thought of Tim. I liked him. He was a good kid. I didn't care where he worked; I just wanted to help him if I could. I figured this could be his big break.

Mom wasn't so sure. "What's he doing here?" she snapped the first time she saw Tim with his recorder. She was even less happy when she found out he was planning to trail me around, sometimes with a photographer.

But Tim was hard not to like: very friendly and polite. Big D bought me a PlayStation while I was at Spaulding—primarily, I think, so he wouldn't have to make conversation. With a PlayStation, Big D and I could trash-talk each other, and neither of us would have to think about my legs. I introduced Tim to my favorite game, *MLB: The Show*. Don't tell the *New York Times*, but we spent hours together playing *The Show*. Of course, he was an intern, so he was probably barely getting paid.

Mom didn't warm up to him, though, until she found out Tim was also raised by a single working mother. And that he had worked his way through college. He had started in engineering, like me, before deciding to take a shot at his dream and switched to journalism.

After that, Mom loved him. Maybe she saw a different version of me in him.

Even now, months later, she asks about him. "So how's Tim doing, Jeff?"

I shake my head. "The worst thing happened to him, Mom. The very worst. The *New York Times* hired him full-time to cover the Mets."

Ha, ha, Tim. Good luck with that. The Mets are terrible.

17.

I read Tim's article about my time at Spaulding recently, and it felt so foreign. The guy in the article seems so sad and alienated. He stares out the window. He answers questions with three words.

He feels like a freak. "There was no escaping all these people," Tim writes, "all their pity and all their questions." In the article, only Erin makes me happy. Or if not happy, at least comfortable.

"Seeing her was the best part of his day now."

I know the article is accurate. Tim spent weeks trailing me, watching everything I did. I look back on all the times I laughed with Michele and other survivors. I remember good times. But I was that guy in the article, too, just wishing everyone would leave me alone. In many ways, I still am. I feel separate from the people around me now, even my family and friends. I feel like they're watching me, like you'd watch a toddler who is happily playing with blocks, but you never know, they could hurl themselves down the stairs at any minute.

It was hard work at Spaulding. Hard work. When my publisher asked me what I wanted people to know after reading the book, one of the things I said was, "I want them to know how hard it was." Moving a two-joint artificial leg, meaning an artificial knee and ankle, takes six times as much strength as moving a regular leg. So I had to get stronger. I had to work myself to exhaustion. Not much is ever accomplished without hard work.

I just wanted to feel normal.

When the photographer, Josh Haner, came to shoot a slideshow presentation for the *New York Times* website, that was what I kept saying: "I just want to be normal." I said it so sadly.

Was I really that morose? There isn't much humor in Tim's article, or in the slideshow. Because they were with me so long, they caught my quiet moments. Those moments were real, but were they the real me?

Maybe that laughing, joking guy wasn't the real me. Maybe I *was* hurting inside.

No, I was *definitely* hurting inside. But the wisecracking patient was me, too, because I never spent much time alone at Spaulding. Erin was usually there, of course, and I could be vulnerable with her. But I had to be "Bauman" for my family, and for the twenty or thirty friends who visited me, including a few people I hadn't seen in years.

There were dozens of strangers, too: cops, EMTs, marathon volunteers, security guards. Carlos came by a few times, and I met the medical tech running alongside him in the iconic photograph. (I still haven't met the woman pushing the wheelchair, Devin Wang, who was a twenty-year-old Boston University student at the time, but I'd like to.) These people were dealing with their own issues, and they needed closure. They needed to feel like we'd won. How could I not meet everyone and tell them how grateful I was?

And how could I seem grateful if I wasn't smiling?

"I'm getting stronger," I told them. "I'm going to feel normal soon."

I felt most comfortable, though, with the other survivors. We were from different economic groups and different parts of the country, but we shared the strongest bond. I don't ever want to see the bloody photographs of the crime scene. But I'd love to see a computer simulation—one of those with the blocky figures that don't even look human—of where all my friends were standing when the bomb exploded. I'd love to get the sense of the moment that brought us together.

I wasn't a fan of our group counseling sessions with the Spaulding psychologist, Dr. Chris Carter. Tim Rohan quoted me as saying the bombers were clowns, but that was only because Dr. Carter asked me. I preferred not to think about the bombers.

And I hated the way people broke down in therapy group. I wanted to be supportive when someone started crying, saying they were depressed and scared, but I also just wanted to get out of there. Of course they were depressed and scared. We all were. I was flipping terrified. The last thing I needed was to hear more about it.

I preferred more informal interactions, like our group workout sessions. There were usually three or four of us on mats in the corner, pulling on lat bars or doing leg lifts with weights tied around our stumps. Once my stomach healed, I did sit-ups and push-ups, both surprisingly difficult without lower legs. My PT Carlyn had to hold my thighs, or I would have tipped backward on every crunch.

My most common workout partners were Patrick and Jess, newlyweds who each lost a leg. I think what they were facing was even harder than what I was going through. I would never trade a missing limb to Erin, even if that meant I'd get a leg back. I'm sure Patrick and Jess would have each lost both limbs if it meant the other could be whole. That's what love is.

But Pat and Jess were so good-natured, always smiling. They never seemed down, even when talking about their difficulties. I was inspired just talking with Pat and Jess about their lives together. Where they were from. What they were like before. What they wanted from their marriage. Pat was a youth pastor, and they both loved Erin, so I think they were hoping to inspire me to propose.

But they weren't above taking the piss, either. In one exercise, I would sit on a cushion and Carlyn would throw a medicine ball to me. I was supposed to catch it without falling over, because walking on artificial legs is all about balance. It was impossible. I'd fall back or to the side every time I caught the ball. And Pat and Jess just laughed at me, calling me Weeble Wobble because I always bounced back up. I mean, it sucked; everything about it sucked. We didn't have much choice but to crack each other up.

The other member of our group, at least for a while, was Ben. He had been hiking in Utah, felt sick, and went to bed. Three months later, he woke up out of a coma with all four of his limbs amputated, all because of a rare bacterial disease. That was so much worse than what I had gone through. That makes no sense.

And yet Ben was the happiest dude. He loved life.

On one side, there's Tamerlan, who grew up in Cambridge. Yes, he was from an immigrant family, and yes, they were poor. But he could have been anything. He had opportunity. And yet he hated life. Hated the world. Hated everyone in it.

On the other side, there's Ben, with no legs or arms, who's smiling every day, just because the sun is shining. And when it's cloudy, he's smiling at the rain.

Then there was Steve, who was clearly struggling. He had lost a leg, but it wasn't his injury that bothered him most. It was the fact that his young son had been beside him. He had seen the blood and felt the heat. He had seen a dead body, and his father injured on the ground. Steve had reached out to him. He had tried to crawl to him, but his son had stared at him, frozen in horror.

And then someone had come and taken him away. They scooped him up, leaving Steve on the ground, unable to move, screaming for his son.

It bothered him. He dwelled on it every day: what his son must have seen, what he must have felt. Steve always looked sad, even when he smiled. Maybe that was how I looked to Tim Rohan when I was lying in my bed, staring out the window at the beautiful spring day, wondering why.

But that was not what I remember most about Steve. I remember the day ALO, my favorite funky California jam band, came to the fifth floor at Spaulding. ALO hadn't played in town since the year before. That will always be a special show, because after the concert, I met Erin. Hard to believe I had only known her for a year.

When my friend Shanette found out ALO was coming back to Boston, she tracked down Zach Gill, their singer, who also played in Jack Johnson's band. She told him about me: how I was a huge fan and had been injured in the bombing.

"Do you think you could stop by and see him?" Shanette asked.

"Sure," Zach said, "but we don't have any transpo to get there."

So Shanette crammed all four band members and two of my other friends in her old Toyota Matrix. We thought the band was just coming to say hello, but they brought their instruments and set up in the fifth-floor visitors' lounge. My friend Kevin O'B. brought a platter of sandwiches from Meat Again and lemonade (no beer in Spaulding), and it was a party.

"Let's get Steve," I said to Shanette. Steve and I had talked about guitar a few times, so I knew he was into music.

Steve came down. ALO jammed. The sun shone through the windows and on the Mystic River outside. I have a video, but about two minutes in the thing turns upside down. Stupid smartphones.

After a while, Zach asked me to jam. My hearing was still bothering me, though, so I said, "Let Steve play for a while."

Steve declined, but you should have seen the smile on his face as he sat in his wheelchair, watching the band. That's what I remember: him looking so happy. When I think about where Steve is now, I imagine him at home, playing with his kid, and that smile on his face.

When I think of Spaulding, that's what I try to think about: the good times. The good friends who made it happen. The good people I met.

But there are other memories, too. Like my first real shower, almost three weeks after the bombing. I turned on the water, expecting a fantastic experience—have you ever gone three weeks without showering? It's awful. But as soon as the water hit my skin, I smelled it: that hellish barbecue on Boylston Street. It was streaming out of my hair and off my skin, like it was coming out of my pores. And suddenly, I was there, lying in the street, on fire. I didn't see the blood, but I felt the terror. My thighs started shaking, and then my whole body started convulsing, like I was having a seizure. I bent down in my shower chair with the hot water running over me and started screaming, without making a sound.

18.

We had two other memorable visitors at Spaulding, a couple of soldiers from the Wounded Warrior Project. I saw plenty of famous people during my recovery: Bradley Cooper; Shawn Thornton from the Bruins; Julian Edelman, Stevan Ridley, and "Gronk" from the Patriots. Dustin Pedroia, Jarrod "Salty" Saltalamacchia, and John Farrell from the Red Sox came by Boston Medical Center and spent one of their rare off days with us.

They were good guys. I liked them a lot. But nobody was more inspiring than those soldiers. And I can't even remember their names! I'm not sure I ever knew them. They were "soldiers," I guess, like I am a "Boston Marathon Survivor."

They had actually visited us before, in the ICU at Boston Medical. I was in such a haze in those days, though, from the drugs and pain, that I don't remember it very well. But I definitely remember them walking into the rehab room at Spaulding during one of our group sessions. I think we all stopped in midstretch, and all the medicine balls fell to the floor. Mine did, anyway. I know walking into a gym doesn't sound like much, but these soldiers had lost both their legs above the knee in combat. They had to have four artificial joints, just like me. And they walked into a room full of people... with confidence... like it was nothing special.

That was what I wanted. I wanted to be able to walk without fear or embarrassment. Up until that moment, I'd never seen it done before.

The soldiers were touring rehabilitation centers, talking with and encouraging people who had lost limbs. It was motivational speaking, I suppose, except they weren't just speaking, they were leading by example.

When they said, "You can do it, Jeff. You can walk," I believed them. I didn't believe my family, or my doctors, or even my therapists. Not entirely. I thought I did, and I wanted to, but there's a difference between thinking something is possible and seeing it in practice.

Those two soldiers made me believe. Because they'd been there, just like me, and they were walking without crutches or even a noticeable limp.

"Give it one year," one of the soldiers told me. "It's hard work, but give it a year and I guarantee you, buddy, you'll be walking."

Those first weeks of rehab are fuzzy. They float in my memory, because of the drugs and the pain. Sometimes, it feels like they never really happened. But I remember those words.

One year.

One year from now, I thought later, alone in my room, means the 2014 Boston Marathon. I had never had a goal. I had dreams and expectations, but nothing specific. I was working, but I wasn't sure exactly what for. Now I saw it.

A chance to give back to Boston.

A chance to show the bombers, on our city's special day, what they had accomplished. Nothing.

At the 2014 Boston Marathon, I was going to walk.

19.

During my second week at Spaulding, Erin had to go back to work. Her office had said she could have a month off, but after three weeks, they realized they needed her. The department was nearing the end of a two-year project, and they couldn't complete it without Erin. She's one of those people whom you don't realize how much she is doing until she's gone.

We had never talked, during those first three weeks, about what Erin needed. I never thought about it, and she didn't want to bother me. I didn't want her to go back to work, for selfish reasons. I can't explain why exactly, but I was afraid to be without her. I told her to stay with me, that I had enough money to support her now, thanks to the generosity of strangers, even if Brigham and Women's fired her.

She told me she wanted to go back. That she needed the routine. Work, she said, would help her eat better and sleep more regularly. She might even get back on her running schedule. She felt run-down and out of shape. She needed a way to help herself so that she'd be able to help me. She was trying to convince herself, I think, as much as me. It was only later that she told me that she cried when her boss told her she had to come back early, and that she spent most of the first week crying at her desk. She never cried around me.

I missed her immediately. As I feared, Spaulding was completely different without Erin. She still spent her evenings with me, but it was hard during the day. She had done all the little things for me: reached for the Kleenex box, picked up the television remote when I dropped it, handed me my guitar when I wanted to play. She knew when to talk, and when I wanted to just lie down. She knew not to ask me if I was okay or if I needed anything. When Mom or Aunt Jenn frustrated me, Erin put her hand on my shoulder. When physical therapy beat me up, Erin helped me into my wheelchair. We even figured out how to lie in bed together, affectionately, without banging my legs. It felt good to feel her body next to mine. I wanted to feel that for the rest of my life.

Erin made me feel comfortable in a way nobody else did. And I needed that, especially then, because I was facing the first big challenge of my public life: a Boston Bruins game.

May was a good month for Boston sports. By May, it had become clear that the Red Sox didn't suck, as expected, and they weren't the cranky, "chicken and beer" malcontents of the past two seasons. They seemed genuinely lovable again, even if they eventually (and inevitably, considering their bullpen) lost their battle for first place with the hated New York Yankees.

The Boston Bruins, our hockey team, were in the playoffs, and of course I'd been watching. I had my Bruins hat and my playoff beard, which I wouldn't shave even for the photo that accompanied the *GQ* article. Erin grumbled about that. She didn't understand. Every hockey fan knows you don't shave during a playoff run.

I hadn't attended a hockey game in twenty years, because the games were so expensive, especially after buying beer, so I wasn't that familiar with the arena traditions. When the Bruins asked me to be the honorary flag captain, I had to ask what that meant. They told me that before each game, a fan was invited onto the ice to wave a Bruins flag, while a huge Bruins banner was handed from section to section around the arena. It pumped up the crowd and got them cheering before the team hit the ice. For the second game of their series against Toronto, the team wanted me to wave the flag.

You might think I'd be thrilled, right? If I was willing to grow a beard for the Bruins, surely I could wave a flag for them.

I said no.

It hurt to sit for more than twenty minutes in my wheelchair, I explained.

I didn't have a way to get to the game.

I hadn't been outside a hospital since the bombing.

That was all true. But really, it all came down to something else: I was scared. I didn't like the idea of being out in public. I felt vulnerable. If another terrorist attack occurred, or if someone targeted me, there was no way I could run. I'd be a sitting target.

And I didn't want anyone to see me. As long as they didn't see me, they could think whatever they wanted about me: that I was a hero, or whatever. I wasn't a hero, though. I was a guy in a wheelchair with no legs. Why would anyone want to see that?

It was one thing to be in Spaulding with other victims. They understood. We could joke about it. But what did the public know? They had legs. They could walk wherever they wanted.

I wasn't like them anymore. And I wasn't like those soldiers at Spaulding. I couldn't walk into a room. I couldn't even stand up. How could I inspire anyone?

"You don't have to do anything you don't want to, Jeff," Erin said. She always told me that: *You don't owe anyone anything. You need to do what's best for your recovery.*

I wanted to be at the game. I wanted to see the Bruins in the playoffs. They were offering me a seat in a luxury box.

And not going…in the end, it felt like chickening out. I didn't want to hide. I had to go out eventually, I told myself, so why not now?

"Will you come with me?" I asked Erin.

"Of course."

That was important, to be with people I trusted. So I talked to the Bruins. They let me bring six people, and that convinced me I could do this. I invited my dad, who was the biggest hockey fan I knew. And his son—my youngest half brother, Alan, who had a weekend off from boot camp. I hadn't seen Alan since the bombing; he'd been in Air Force boot camp when it happened. Because of the strict rules of boot camp, we'd barely even talked on the phone. Big D came, too, of course, and Sully, Erin, and my cousin Mary Kate, Uncle Bob's daughter.

We received a police escort from Spaulding to the TD Garden. It was only a mile, but the traffic was thick. I sat in my wheelchair, in my Bruins jersey, staring out the window at all the other fans in black and gold. I could see a few drivers craning their necks as the police escort nudged them onto the shoulder, and a few more cursing at us. Typical Boston. Even though I was in a handicapped van, they probably thought I was a politician.

"I'm not going on the ice," I said.

"Come on, son," my dad said.

Erin squeezed my hand. "It's all right," she whispered.

I had told the Bruins this might happen. *I haven't been outside since the bombing*, I'd explained. *I'm screwed up. I can't guarantee anything.*

They said they understood, but I knew I was letting them down. I tried to think my way through my fear, but the more I thought about the crowded arena, the more I felt trapped. It was like being on the high dive…in front of a crowd…in my wheelchair. Staring down at the water wasn't going to help. I wasn't even comfortable with the idea of sitting in a private box.

I probably should have practiced being outside, I thought. I probably should have spent time around people I didn't know to see how it felt. But there was no way I could back out now.

"I can't do it," I said again. "I'll watch the game, but I can't go out there."

We reached the arena and pulled into the loading dock next to the ambulances. There was a short ramp, and then we were so close to the ice you could feel the chill. The public relations people for the Bruins were waiting. I had told them no media and no interviews, so it was a small group.

"Are you ready?" they asked me.

"Let's do this thing," I said.

I still don't know why. It was just... when I got into the arena, I suddenly felt like I could do it. No, that I *should* do it. And most important, that I *wanted* to do it.

They handed me a huge flag, about six feet across. Erin pushed me to the mouth of the tunnel. I chatted with the Bruins people, trying not to look at the crowd across the ice. Breathe, Jeff, I told myself. You can do this.

Then the lights went out completely, and the music started pumping. I couldn't see a thing as Erin rolled me along a carpet over the ice. It was pitch-black, until words started appearing on the Jumbotron overhead:

By now you all know his inspirational story
His perseverance in the face of great adversity
represents all that is...
BOSTON
(flash, flash)
STRONG

The arena lights came on, and I started waving the flag like crazy. I just kept waving and waving, trying not to look around. It felt like I was at the bottom of the ocean. The crowd rose up and up, climbing away from me into the shadows, but their enthusiasm wasn't scary. It was contagious. I pumped a fist, and a huge cheer rolled over me. It was like being onstage at a concert. I swung the flag as high as I could. It tangled around the pole, and Erin stepped up to untangle it for me. The crowd didn't stop. They cheered louder. I pumped my fist for them, a huge smile on my face. Usually, the flag says Bruins. This one said Boston Strong.

They weren't just cheering for the team. They were cheering for our city.

People kept coming up to me in the private box afterward, wanting to shake my hand. The whole game, people kept slapping me on the back, telling me how proud they were. In the van on the way over, that would have terrified me: strangers, backslapping, a screaming crowd. But in the moment, it felt right. These people weren't staring at me. They weren't expecting anything. They just wanted to let me know they cared.

20.

A few days after the game, Kevin took me out to lunch. He was back at Costco, but he still checked in with me every day and often came by. This was only my second time out of the hospital; I think Kevin had to talk the nurses into letting me go. Kevin is good at talking people into things.

We went to Flour, one of the restaurants that had given my family and me free meals when I was at BMC. I transferred from the car to the wheelchair with ease, and the owner treated us to a cart full of food. Afterward, Kevin took me for a haircut. Ever since the shower, I had hated my hair. The 'fro had to go. I was allowed to be away for only two hours, but that was enough. I hadn't brought any pain medicine with me. By the time we got back to Spaulding, my legs and back were sore from sitting so long in my wheelchair.

By then, I knew I would be discharged. Most patients stayed in Spaulding for at least two weeks after receiving their artificial legs, but I had already been in hospitals for a month. I badgered my doctors to send me home, and I even enlisted the help of my physical therapist, Carlyn. Behind the scenes, Erin was working just as hard to get me home. She knew how much the Island of Misfit Toys affected me. Even in Spaulding, with my fellow survivors, I felt like I was on display. My doctors finally agreed that as soon as my stomach incision healed, I could transition to outpatient care, as long as I agreed to come in for physical therapy four times a week.

On my last day, Carlyn asked if I wanted to try a special workout. Spaulding had several boats and kayaks that could be launched from behind the building, and Carlyn thought the kayak would be perfect for me.

Michele, Remy, and me with our marathon swag, just before leaving for the finish line. This was the last photo taken before all three of us were injured in the bombing. *(Photo courtesy of Remy Lawler)*

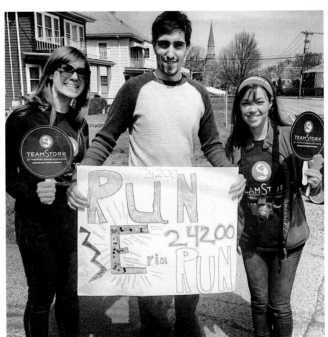

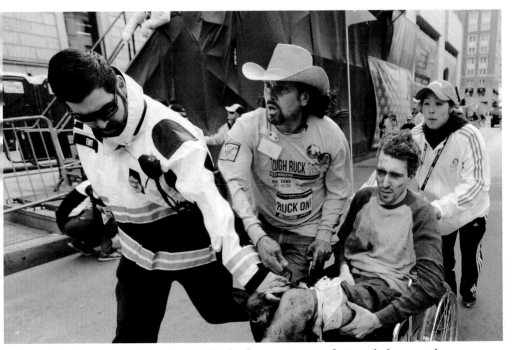

The famous bombing photo. I think of it as a picture of triumph, because three people are saving my life. But I still don't like to look at it. *(AP Photo/Charles Krupa)*

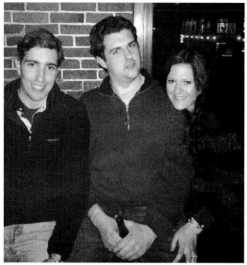

Big D, Aunt Jenn, and me at Erin's Team Stork fundraiser on April 1, 2013, only two weeks before the bombing. *(Photo courtesy of Jenn Joyce Maybury)*

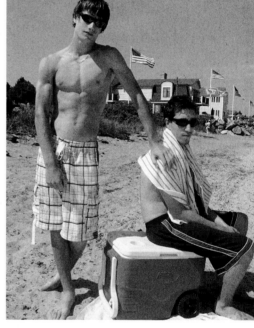

My half-brother Alan and me at the beach in Seabrook, New Hampshire, in 2011. *(Photo courtesy of Alan G. Bauman)*

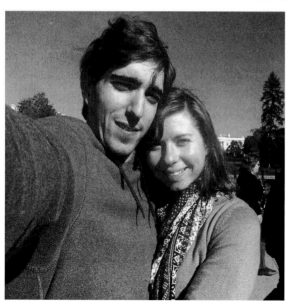

Erin and me in the fall of 2012. This photo hung on my IV while I was in the intensive care unit at Boston Medical Center. *(Photo courtesy of Erin Hurley)*

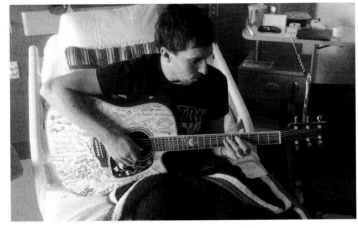

Playing one of my donated guitars at Spaulding. I couldn't hear the notes very well because of damage to my inner ears, but look at the signatures! *(Photo courtesy of Jenn Joyce Maybury)*

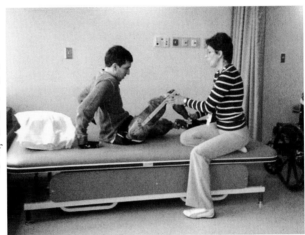

My physical therapist, Michelle Kerr, works on my right leg during a session at Spaulding. Believe me: It usually wasn't this gentle. *(Photo courtesy of Jenn Joyce Maybury)*

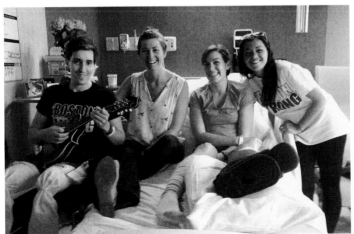

One of Erin's favorite photos: the two of us with her best friends, Remy and Michele. This was taken in Michele's room at Spaulding, about three weeks after the bombing. *(Photo courtesy of Remy Lawler)*

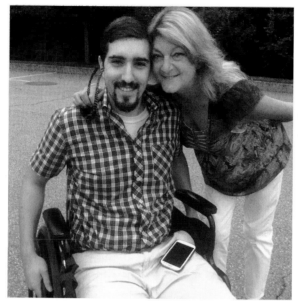

Mom and me. *(Photo courtesy of Jenn Joyce Maybury)*

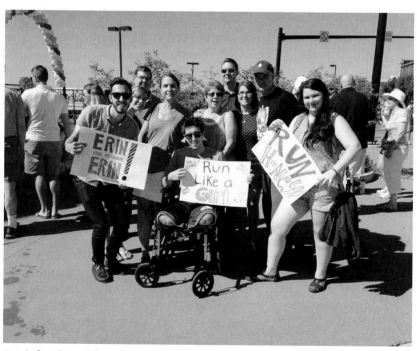

Erin's family and friends, including Remy and Michele, at the Portsmouth Half Marathon in Maine. It was tough being in the crowd, but we did it for Erin. *(Photo courtesy of Gail Goodson)*

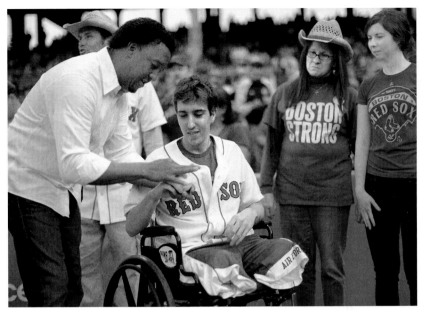

My childhood idol, Pedro Martinez, demonstrates how he grips a changeup, while Erin and Carlos's wife Mel look on. He surprised me on the field at Fenway before my first pitch on May 28, 2013. *(Credit: Josh Haner/The New York Times/ Redux)*

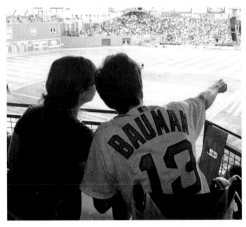

Relaxing with my E. a few innings later. I wouldn't have been there without her. *(Photo courtesy of Jenn Joyce Maybury)*

Game 2 of the World Series at Fenway with two great friends I made during my recovery: Tim Rohan and Katlyn (Kat) Townsend. Sorry the Mets didn't make it, Tim. Maybe next decade. *(Photo courtesy of Katlyn Townsend)*

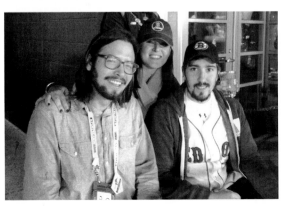

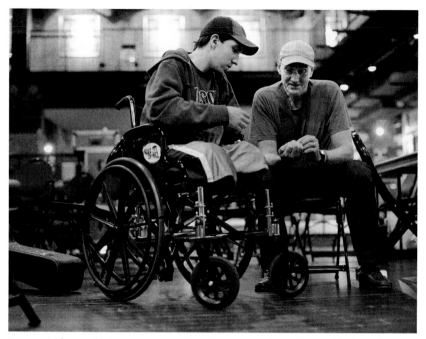

James Taylor took the time to really talk to me at his rehearsal before the One Fund concert. A truly caring dude. *(Credit: Josh Haner/The* New York Times/ *Redux)*

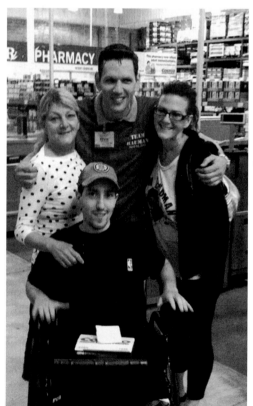

With Mom, Aunt Jenn, and Kevin "Heavy Kevy" Horst during my first visit to the Costco where I worked. *(Photo courtesy of Jenn Joyce Maybury)*

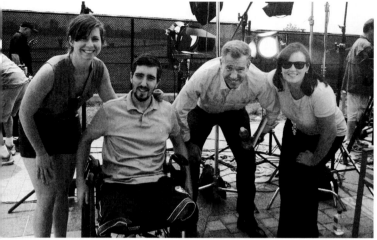

Erin, Kat, and me with Brian Williams after my only national television interview in July 2013. *(Photo courtesy of Katlyn Townsend)*

Carlos Arredondo and three generations of Jeffs: me, my dad Big Jeff, and my great-uncle Jeff. *(Photo courtesy of Terri Wright Bauman)*

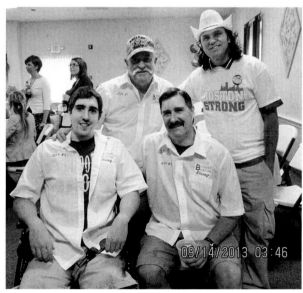

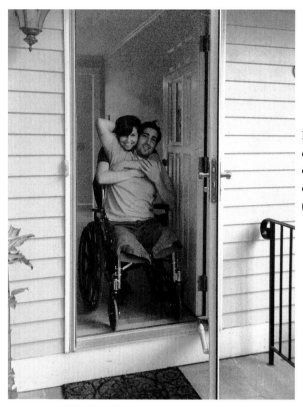

Erin and me on our first day in our new home—and our new lives. Now shut the door, Mom. Bauman out! *(Photo courtesy of Kevin Horst)*

Here we are today, with the love of our lives, Nora Gail Bauman, born July 13, 2014. *(Josh Haner/ The New York Times/Redux)*

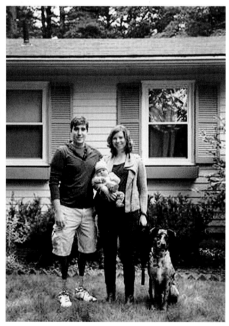

So around 10:00 in the morning, Carlyn and I slipped into two kayaks, then into the Mystic River. Boat therapy is common in Boston, and I can see why. Uncle Bob had often taken me out in his bass boat on the Concord River, sometimes floating all the way to the Old North Bridge, where the first battle of the Revolutionary War was fought, but there was nothing like being in a kayak in the middle of the city. The boat just glides along the water beneath you as the warehouses slip past, and with no need for legs, it was almost possible to stop missing mine. It wasn't long before we were rounding the point into the harbor. I was hoping to paddle next to a freighter, but there were only small boats on the water that morning.

Once in the harbor, we headed south, toward downtown. Before long, I could see the three spires and sails of the USS *Constitution*, the oldest ship in the United States Navy. Commissioned in 1794 and named by George Washington, it had been a symbol of Boston for almost a hundred years. We paddled toward it until it towered over us, and although we couldn't get close enough to touch it, because of barriers in the water to protect it from people like me, it still felt like I was touching Boston history.

I slipped out of Spaulding a few days later, on May 17, 2013, one month and two days after the bombing. My family had argued for weeks about where I would go. My dad wanted me with him in New Hampshire. Uncle Bob and Aunt Jenn wanted me to move in with them. They never said it outright, but they were worried about Mom. She had been handling herself well, but what if a crisis occurred? What if I fell, or needed quick medical attention? Mom wasn't good in a crisis. And everyone was worried about her stress.

Erin couldn't believe that I was caught in the middle of it. "This drama isn't good for you," she'd say.

I didn't think anything of it. My family had always been like that. They cared for each other so much that they couldn't help but argue, and they tried to help so much that they always got in each other's way.

"What does Jeff want?" Erin always said, whenever they asked her opinion. "That's the only thing that matters. It's his life."

If I had my choice, and my legs, I'd have moved in with Erin. But she lived on the second floor of a classic Boston triple decker—a three-story house with an apartment on each floor. The stairs were rickety and uneven, and they curved around a corner. I knew there was no way I'd ever go in that apartment again.

In the end, there was no drama at all. I decided to go back to Mom's for a few weeks, as I always knew I would, while Erin and I looked into getting an apartment together. The media loved reporting when survivors left the hospital, but I kept my leaving quiet. There was no media coverage, no party, and no sad good-byes, especially since I'd be back four days a week for therapy. Uncle Bob and Aunt Cathleen pulled up to the door, threw my wheelchair in the trunk, and we were gone, just the three of us, with Tim Rohan and Josh Haner from the *New York Times* following in their own car.

About ten miles down the road, Uncle Bob noticed we were being followed. I wasn't listed in any directories, and we were keeping my home address a secret. I didn't like the idea of media waiting for me, as they had been in Aunt Jenn's driveway once when she came home from visiting me in the hospital. I didn't want to worry that some nut-jobs would be outside my front door with a rifle, saying, "This guy is a symbol. If we take him out, we send a message."

So Uncle Bob called a friend in the Chelmsford police department about our dilemma, and I have to admit, he seemed to enjoy the conversation.

"It's taken care of," he said.

And he was right. Just outside Chelmsford, there was a huge banner hanging from the highway overpass: WELCOME HOME JEFF. BAUMAN STRONG.

"Your aunt Cathleen never could keep a secret." Uncle Bob laughed.

And just beyond the sign was a police cruiser. As soon as we passed, the sirens came on, and the car following us was pulled over. Apparently, the occupants were from a national news organization, and the officer had a nice time interrogating them, especially when Tim and Josh went cruising past.

"But that's the *New York Times*," one of them complained.

"I'm sorry, ma'am. I'd like to help you, but I can't pull someone over just because they work for the *New York Times*."

He delayed them for only a minute, but it was enough to get us home.

21.

There was a fund-raiser for me that night at the Chelmsford Radisson, organized by Sully and his sister. It was a raffle and dance, with a pay bar, in the big banquet room at the hotel. It was a coincidence that it fell on the night I arrived home; Sully and Brooke had been planning it for a month. No one, including my doctors, expected me home so soon.

I intended to make an appearance. People kept calling me, and I kept telling them I would be there. But I didn't want to go. I'd been pushing myself hard to get home; it was a huge moment when I rolled through the door and into our living room–kitchen. (It's a three-room apartment.) After spending a month trying to get home, the last thing I wanted to do was leave.

I was tired. Really tired. And in that condition, or maybe any condition, I had no desire to see everyone I'd ever known. There were four hundred people at the fund-raiser, Sully told me. They were serving Bauman Bionic Brew. I had to see it. The label was a picture of my face on the body of Iron Man. People wanted to toast me. They wanted to say hi. But the more excited they were to see me, home and well, the less excited I became.

"Just say no," Erin said when I called her for advice. "They never planned for you to come, anyway."

But I couldn't say no. And when I hedged—"I'm tired, guys"—they wouldn't take the hint. My friends kept calling.

"We miss you, bro."

"It's a party."

"Bauman always shows up for a party."

About halfway through, my dad came by the apartment. He wouldn't come into Mom's apartment, where he knew he wasn't welcome. He stood in front of the building and tried to convince me to put in an appearance.

"I'll drive you," he said. "It will be easy."

He didn't understand. Nothing was easy.

Finally, around eleven, I lay down in my own bed for the first time in a month and tried, unsuccessfully, to fall asleep.

The next morning, Mom called my brother Tim. Tim's a plumber, has been for years. He had become friends with the Odoms in the hospital, and Mr. Odom, who owned a mechanical contracting business in California, was helping him finally get into the pipefitter's union. The circle of kindness, you know. It keeps going on.

"You need to get over here," Mom told Tim. "Jeff wants to take a shower, but he can't reach the knobs. He needs one of those handheld shower nozzles."

"Ah, Ma, I told you he was going to need that last week." It was obvious Tim wasn't feeling too good. "Okay," he muttered, when Mom wouldn't let it go. "I'll come over this afternoon."

"No, Tim, you gotta get over here now. Your brother needs you."

Tim showed up a half hour later. He looked like hell, and he was hopping on one foot. He couldn't even put his right foot on the ground.

"We went to the Hong Kong after the party," he admitted. "Vinnie gave us free drinks. For Bow-Man, he said. The whole place was toasting you. Bow-man! Bow-man! I tripped on a sprinkler head coming out."

"Sniper on the roof!" I yelled, imagining Tim going down like he'd been shot. I still say that to Tim whenever I see him. "Sniper on the roof!"

Like I said before, nothing good ever happens in the Hong Kong.

The next day, Tim's lower leg was a balloon. Turns out he'd broken his foot the week before, when he dropped a cast-iron bathtub on it. He'd tweaked the break when he tripped outside the Hong Kong.

But he came through for me, like he always did. He installed the handheld, and that afternoon, in Mom's apartment, I took my first pain-free shower since losing my legs.

———————

The sutures holding my thighs together came out a few days later. "Compared to everything else you've been through, this will be a breeze," my surgeon, Dr. Kalish, told me in the exam room at Boston Medical Center.

I didn't believe him. My legs looked bad. These weren't stitches, they were metal wires, and most of them were covered with bloody masses that looked like boils. I made the mistake of checking on them the day I got home. I immediately texted Dr. Kalish a few photographs. He said, yes, they were infected, but don't worry, he'd take care of them when the sutures came out.

Now here he was, telling me not to worry again, before leaving me with a resident, who raised her pliers, smiled nervously, and said, "Ready?"

I lay back on the table and stared out the window. An American flag was flying at half-staff. I thought about Martin, Krystle, and Lingzi Lu, who had all died at the bombing. And Officer Sean Collier, who had been sitting in his patrol car when the bombers snuck up from behind and shot him five times, twice in the head. I wondered if the flag was for the victims of the bombing, or if the hospital had moved on. Had another tragedy occurred? Or did the flag often fly that way? Surely someone died at Boston Medical Center every day.

By the time those thoughts had crossed my mind, I was crying. I gritted my teeth against the pain and felt the tears rolling down my cheeks. I wanted the resident to be finished, but sometimes, when she yanked hard, I cried out, and she stopped.

"Oh, okay. Do you need a break?"

I shook my head no. Dr. Kalish came back to finish me off. There were ten deep sutures that needed a surgical hand. I whimpered, according to Tim Rohan in his *New York Times* piece, as Dr. Kalish tugged and jerked the wires through my skin. I stared at the flag, flying at half-staff. It looked like a storm was coming.

Then it was over.

Dr. Kalish wiped the blood off his instruments, shook my hand, and said, "You did it. I hope that wasn't so awful."

Or as Tim put it: "After this, there would be no more procedures. There was nothing more his doctors could do. His legs would be this way for the rest of his life. Learning to walk again, and whatever happened after that, was up to him."

Poetry. Pure bandbox poetry. But you can save it for Matt Harvey's elbow, son.

I'm walking.

WALKING

22.

I was hoping to be measured for my artificial legs at BMC the day my sutures came out, but after the operation I was too bloody and sore. So two days later, Mom drove me to United Prosthetics in Dorchester, a south Boston neighborhood. The company had been founded in 1914 by Philip Martino, an immigrant from Italy who was trained as a shoemaker. That's what their website said anyway.

Paul Martino, Philip Martino's grandson, told me a slightly longer story. He said his grandfather actually started carving wooden legs in his kitchen in 1903. He carved every leg by hand for a specific patient, then wrapped the wood in leather and provided a leather cable to hold it in place. Two of his customers liked their new legs so much, the three of them went into business together. They eventually received a government contract to provide artificial legs to soldiers wounded in World War I, and they had been a fixture in Boston ever since.

It was cool, listening to this guy talk about the company. I could tell he loved his family, and he loved fake legs. It was even cooler when he pointed at a shelf, and there they were: real pirate-style wooden legs that old-timers had actually used. The office wasn't fancy. It was in a nondescript industrial area and looked like an old police barracks. But it had history. It was like a museum of legs in there.

"This is your leg," Mr. Martino said. "The Genium."

Mr. Martino had come to Spaulding a few weeks before to give me my shrinkers, tight cotton mesh socks designed to shape the ends of my legs. The shrinkers were so tight they pushed some of my sutures into my thigh, making their removal more painful, but it was a necessary step. Legs become sensitive after they've been blown apart; they couldn't have handled the pressure of the sockets otherwise.

During that visit, Mr. Martino showed me the Genium. The manufacturer, Ottobock, had agreed to donate my pair, and the installation was being covered by donations. "We had a lot of calls from concerned citizens," Mr. Martino told me. "They told us to make sure that kid gets the best. These are the best."

Still, actually holding the thing was intimidating. The Genium wasn't wooden, and it wasn't one of those legs that's plastic and flesh-colored, so at first you don't notice it, until something sticks in your mind as not quite right, and you do a double take.

The Genium looked like a Terminator leg. I mean that part at the end of the first movie, when you think Arnold Schwarzenegger is burned up in the tanker explosion, but then he comes out with just his metal skeleton, and they show his legs clanking along, with motor sounds, like nothing could stop them. The Genium was metal and plastic, with a titanium joint and a metal plate that attached to my socket—the part that would slip over my thigh—with four industrial-size bolts. Nothing about it seemed human. It had steel rails and a metal pole for adjusting your height and what looked like a piston hidden behind a plastic shin, which moved as the leg bent. Etched on the front, like the brand on a bicycle, were the words: Genium Bionic Prosthetic System.

Holy cow, I thought. These legs really are bionic.

And it was heavy, at least when the six-inch-long central component was attached to the thigh socket and the foot. It was so heavy it was hard to lift with one arm.

"The technology was developed by the government for soldiers during Operation Desert Storm," Mr. Martino explained. "It was improved during the invasions in Iraq and Afghanistan. A lot of people lost limbs over there. They're a hundred grand a leg, but the public demanded the best."

What about other people? I wondered. What about car crash victims? What about hikers like Ben, who wake up to find all their limbs gone? Ben had never been in the news. Who was paying his bills?

Mr. Martino explained how the legs worked. I listened intently, but most of it went over my head. I caught that the pistons were hydraulic tubes filled with fluid. They weren't meant to lift the leg. They were created to slow your descent if you fell, so that you wouldn't go straight down and break your tailbone.

"Are you okay?" Erin asked, putting a hand on my shoulder.

"Yes, why?"

"You're rubbing your thighs again."

I looked down. I was digging the heel of my hands into my thighs and pushing down toward the ends of my legs. It was a habit. My legs always hurt, and rubbing them made them feel better. It also calmed my nerves.

The knees, Mr. Martino said, contained a microchip to control the hydraulics. (Robot legs!) The microchip processed information one hundred times a second, through six sensors built into the knee unit. That wasn't nearly as fast as your spine processed information—because walking and balancing aren't brain functions, they are spine functions—but far faster than any previous artificial leg. Again, though, all this technology didn't help you bend your knees or move them faster. That was the responsibility of your muscles. It was designed to keep your legs balanced and your foot level, especially on uneven ground.

I was starting to see a pattern here. These legs may have looked like parts of a motorcycle, but they weren't the engine. They were the kickstand. Everything was geared toward not falling down.

"Any questions?"

Only a million. Like: Why does so much have to go into staying upright? Is it that difficult? If this is twenty years of technology, why isn't it more like Iron Man?

"No, I've got it."

"Good. Then let's fit you for some sockets."

Mr. Martino measured my thighs. Then he wrapped them in plastic and netting. He covered the netting with strips of plaster, sort of like how you make a papier-mâché mask for a science project in school. The plaster would form molds. The molds would then be used to shape hard plastic sockets that would fit tightly over each leg. The molds needed to be as exact as possible. My thighs were my only leg muscles now; they had to press on the socket to lift the rest of the leg. The more snugly the socket fit, the less effort would be wasted, and the more comfortable movement would feel.

I lay back and tried not to think about the complexity. All the things that could go wrong. I thought of the two soldiers who had visited me at Spaulding. The way they walked right into the room, like it was nothing.

The way they said, "You can do it, Jeff."

Ten months. That was how long I had until the next Boston Marathon. I didn't have any doubt: I'd be walking by then.

"Trust the leg." That was what Mr. Martino said. "You have to trust the leg. That's the most important thing."

Okay, Pops. I got you. I'm ready to go.

23.

It would take about a week to manufacture my socket. I spent most of that time at home, except for my appointments. I still had checkups at BMC and physical therapy at Spaulding. Since I couldn't drive, and Erin was working, Mom took me. It was good to see all my new friends, but the exercises were brutal, especially now that I had a new physical therapist, Michelle Kerr, who specialized in prosthetics. My left leg was weaker than my right, and that was a problem.

"How do I balance them?" I asked her.

"You work both of them harder."

It was more of the same: leg lifts, sit-ups, push-ups. I was strong enough now to hold myself in a crunch position with my legs lifted, so Michelle gave me a medicine ball and made me turn side to side, working my abs. I rode the arm bicycle, a stationary bike with the pedals on the handlebars, to work on my cardio and endurance. I strapped weights to my thighs and lifted them in all directions. It was tough. Michelle had been working with amputees for years; she knew how to push. I couldn't even walk after some of those workouts, I was so sore.

Just kidding. I couldn't walk, anyway.

Seriously, though, I would leave so sore I couldn't sit without pain. I'd grit my teeth and shift my weight the whole hour home, trying not to let Mom know how much it hurt.

When I wasn't exercising, I was usually at Mom's apartment, trying to sleep. My body craved rest. It was begging me to stop moving, to just lie down and heal. But for a month, I hadn't been able to sleep. My mind was too lit up. The nurses gave me Xanax once, and I went to sleep, but half an hour later I was sitting bolt upright in bed with my eyes open, unresponsive but agitated. They never tried that again.

It was more of the same at home: lying in bed with my mind spinning, or snapping awake in a hot sweat, unsure of where I was. But at least at home, I had space. I could be alone, without anyone prodding me or asking questions. That first week, I'd lie in a semi-aware state for hours, trying to remain calm, trying to let my body recover. I was on a lot of pain medication. I was physically beat. I probably spent sixteen hours a day in bed, although I'd only sleep for three or four. I'd stare at the ceiling, thinking: You're done with the hospital, Jeff. You're free.

But I wasn't done. And I wasn't free.

I could see that as soon as the first light crept through my blinds every morning. My first thought was always to stand up and walk. No, I wouldn't even think it. I'd just do it, like I had every morning for twenty-seven years. Then I'd realize there was nothing to swing over the edge of the bed, and no way to touch the ground.

I'd roll onto my back in my sweaty covers. I was always sweaty, no matter how cool it was in the apartment. I'd think, Go to sleep, Jeff. Just go to sleep and forget all this.

My room was a Hobbit hole, ten-by-ten, with only one small window. When I'd left for the marathon, it was mostly empty. Clothes were scattered everywhere, and my guitar was in the corner, but otherwise I had only a twin bed, a dresser, and one chair. Now I'd roll over in bed and see a room crammed full of guitars and a mandolin, a pile of stuffed animals and gear saying Bruins, Red Sox, Boston Strong. My dresser was covered with letters, photos, and cards. I had so many new shirts, they wouldn't fit in my drawers. I piled them on my chair, since I couldn't reach the hangers in my closet. It was shirts on top, shorts underneath, socks in a drawer. I had a system. I don't want you to think I'm a slob.

I have to get up, I'd think. I have to keep going.

I couldn't do crunches at home. It was hard to get down on the floor, and I'm not sure there was enough space anyway. But I could do arm exercises, stretches, and core work.

Eventually, I'd roll into the living room, and Mom would be there, sitting at the table where she displayed her photographs. Derek and me at a Sox game when I was six years old. Me in my junior hockey uniform. Forehead's first-grade school picture. My high school portrait, one of those casual ones where I'm wearing jeans and my shirt is untucked. For some reason, I'm not wearing shoes or socks. It was a reminder that not so long ago, I had feet.

But now, behind the usual photos, was a huge framed "get well" photo signed by all the employees at my Costco. Cards were propped in every extra inch. The space under the table was packed with gifts, like hand-sewn blankets and orange guitar amps, and mementos, like the two wooden transfer boards I'd used to get into my wheelchair in the hospital. I hadn't needed them for weeks, but Mom couldn't part with them.

In one corner, three paper grocery bags were filled with cards and letters.

"That's not all of them," Mom told me. "There's more at your aunt Jenn's house. We're sorting and keeping every one of them, for when you're ready."

Mom was still off work, still trying to care for me. I didn't like to be cared for, but there were so many things I couldn't do. I couldn't reach the top half of the refrigerator; I couldn't grab things on the stove. The corner outside my bedroom was tight, and sometimes I needed help getting my wheelchair through. The hospital sent occupational therapists to show me how to arrange the apartment and manage everyday functions, but after two visits I told them not to come back. It was a waste of money. Mom and I could figure things out on our own.

So Mom spent much of the day running errands for me or helping with simple tasks. We didn't talk much, but that wasn't new. I had always kept my emotions to myself. Instead of chatting—instead of working through things that way—Mom read my mail. She kept the special notes to show to me and took a few very special ones each day and stuck them on the refrigerator. Often, these were the notes that made her cry.

"Why do you do that to yourself, Mom?"

"Because they took the time, Jeffrey."

And because they made her happy. Even when she cried.

I feel bad sometimes about not reading all the letters. They were an important part of my recovery. It was empowering to know that so many people cared. It motivated me.

But reading the letters overwhelmed me, too. People wrote to say they were naming workout routines after me, or that I helped them deal with their grief over a personal tragedy, or that their small city in Wisconsin felt safer because of me.

How could that be? I didn't feel safer.

Elementary school children drew me pictures. Kindergarten classrooms wrote stories about me. Tim's wife, Erika, was a kindergarten teacher in Lowell, and her class made a big banner, and each child wrote me a personal message. She said it helped the children understand the bombing and feel less afraid.

I wanted to send them all a PlayStation. I really did. I just wanted to give it all back. But I could see why, as Mom told me in the hospital, that wasn't possible. There was no way to give back to everyone who had given to me.

So please know, especially if you wrote to me and never heard back, that I loved the letters. They motivated me when I didn't want to get out of bed. But more than that, they helped my mom.

She had been through hell. She had seen her son with his legs blown off, and she had spent a day thinking I might die. She had sat for days in my hospital room, then driven home and sat for hours alone in her apartment, exhausted and afraid. But she was strong. She never gave in to despair. She cried, and she worried, but she always believed the fighter in me would win through.

I'm not saying Mom didn't deserve the concern of her brother and sisters. Mom was fragile. She struggled. She drank, sometimes too much. When she was sober, I loved her. She was a good person.

Even when she had been drinking too much, she was never mean. She was *emotional*. It was like she couldn't contain her disappointments, and she had to talk them out, with anger and tears. She had to give me advice and tell me what to do. She wasn't insulting me. She was nagging. She so desperately wanted me to be happy, to be successful, that she couldn't stop herself. To be honest, even though we lived together, we hadn't seen much of each other in years. Mom worked during the day, and I tried to stay out with friends or family at night.

But in the weeks after my injury, Mom stayed away from the wine. She stayed away from pity. Small setbacks can be unbearable, but big disasters . . . a lot of people, like Mom, find strength in those moments.

And she had the letters.

They weren't for her. If Mom ever received a thank-you or a note of encouragement, she didn't share it with me. She didn't care. Through this whole ordeal, she has never asked for anything. People in Concord, New Hampshire, donated supplies and labor to remodel my dad's house. They built a new wheelchair-accessible deck, a new first-floor bedroom, even a new kitchen. Mom got a two-foot ramp and a wider bathroom door.

Anything else, I think, she would have found insulting. What? Are you saying the apartment I've spent twenty years waitressing double-shifts to pay for isn't good enough?

When I told her I wanted to buy her something with the donations, she refused. I said it again and again, and she always refused. "That money is for you and Erin," she said. "For your medical bills. And your children. As long as you're taken care of, Jeffrey, I don't care if I live in a paper bag."

I went to the fridge and pulled out a bottle of Cavit wine. "Here you go," I said, handing her the paper bag she always kept her wine in.

Don't get me wrong, Mom drove me crazy. She worried, and she treated me like a child. She knocked on my door every half hour, it seemed. "Jeff, are you all right?"

"Yes, Mom." *I'm lying on my bed, massaging my thigh, hoping this mind-shattering pain will work its way out of my muscles, but I'm fine.*

I guess what I'm trying to say is...when I needed her, Mom was there. All my life, she is the one who has been there for me. And I don't know if I ever tell her, but I love her for it. I love her for who she is.

So thank you, Mom.

We made it. Together.

24.

The Red Sox had called me weeks ahead of time to discuss throwing out the first pitch. Say what you will about the franchise, all you haters, but they had embraced their role as Boston's team, and they had dedicated their season to honoring first responders and victims of the bombing. Heather Abbott, who was injured in the bombing, was the first to throw a pitch in early May. Seven family members of Sean Collier, the police officer killed on the Thursday after the bombing, would end the tributes in late August.

I was in the middle. I needed to be healed enough to throw without pain, so we settled on May 28—a little more than six weeks after the bombing. At that time, the bullpen was in trouble. Two players were hurt, and they had just elevated a thirty-eight-year-old Japanese dude to be the closer. I think we were all anticipating a dive in the standings, but May 28 turned out to be the day the Sox moved ahead of the Yankees for good.

Big D and I went out the morning of the game to practice pitching in the parking lot outside Mom's apartment. Throwing out the first pitch is a great baseball tradition. I mean, United States presidents do it. I'd seen enough people botch it, though, to know it wasn't as easy as it seemed. Especially from a wheelchair. Fortunately, I figured out how to turn myself at an angle for maximum velocity just before we lost the baseball in the poison ivy.

Yo, Big D. I have a limited catching area. Don't make me jump for a high throw.

The Sox said I could invite as many people as I wanted, so we had eight people waiting outside Mom's when the team limousine pulled up.

They had a personalized jersey for me with "Bauman" on the back. I immediately put it on. Underneath, where no one could see it, I had on a Captain America shirt that someone had given me.

We hit traffic on the way in, so we arrived late. The Red Sox rushed us straight from the players' parking lot to the groundskeeper's area along the first base line. I could hear cameras clicking, and I saw fans getting their hot dogs and beers stop in their tracks. Some of them started clapping.

"Way to go, Jeff," someone said.

"Thank you," others yelled.

I waved back as we hustled along. At the edge of the field, Carlos was waiting in his trademark cowboy hat, along with a security detail. He smiled when he saw me and gave me a hug. It was our first public appearance together, although I'd seen him several times at the hospital. He looked good in his "Arredondo" jersey—smiling, friendly, shaking everyone's hand. He had taken some flak from the press because he'd been making a lot of public appearances since the bombing, but as his wife, Mel, pointed out, he had been making public appearances on behalf of the troops for years. That was what he did with his life. There was just more press covering those appearances now.

This was only my second time in public, and my first with Carlos, so the Sox were making a big deal out of it—"the hero and his hero." They had asked me if there was anyone I wanted to pitch to, so of course I chose my personal hero, the greatest pitcher in Red Sox history, Roger "The Rocket" . . .

Nah. Come on.

I wanted Pedro, the greatest Red Sox pitcher of all time. Back in the late 1990s and early 2000s, when I was a teenager, Pedro Martinez was the undisputed best pitcher in the world. He was the star of some lean years, and he was still a star when the Sox won the World Series for the first time in eighty-six years in 2004. Uncle Bob had season tickets that year, and Big D and I were there for Game 4, when the Sox tied it in the ninth, and Big Papi hit the game-winning homer in the twelfth to start the greatest series comeback in baseball history.

Pedro was retired, but he still worked for the Sox. Unfortunately, he was out of town that day, so I had to go with my second choice, Jarrod "Salty" Saltalamacchia, the Red Sox starting catcher. Salty wasn't one of the best players on the team. In fact, at that point, he was hanging on to his starting job primarily because David Ross was hurt. He was a dirt dog, though, a scrapper, always hustling and studying. He was my kind of player, but he'd never been my favorite.

The reason I chose him was because he had come to the hospital after the bombing. I'd been doing local charity events for months, and it's funny how often you see the same people. Shawn Thornton from the Bruins. Jenny Dell, the local station sideline reporter. Clay Buchholz and Salty from the Sox. When you meet people, you can tell if they're solid. That was the way it was with Salty. If this Red Sox team was built on character, as everyone was saying, then it was built on players like Salty. He wasn't a star, but he was a good guy.

"Awesome to see you again, Jeff," he said when I met him on the field.

Carlos had chosen Big Papi, so I shook his hand as well.

It was surreal. We were on the field at Fenway, chatting with Salty and Papi, while thousands cheered. Thousands. I didn't think it could get any better, until someone came up behind me and tapped me on the shoulder.

I turned around. It was Pedro.

"What . . . what are you doing here?" I managed to say.

"I came to see you, buddy," he said.

We started talking. Pedro was funny, like he'd always been on television. I was so nervous, but chatting with Pedro calmed me down. I asked him for advice on my pitch, and he showed me how to grip his fastball. Then he showed me the changeup.

Someone came over and said it was time. I looked up, and Pedro and I were surrounded by cameras. I was near the fence, and I noticed people in the front row reaching toward me. They wanted my autograph. I started signing as fast as I could, trying to talk with everyone, and I remember looking over, a big smile on my face, and Erin giving me a thumbs-up.

Maybe those people remember meeting me. I hope they do. Because you know what I remember? Meeting them. I remember seeing them so happy, especially the kids. I would have signed autographs all day.

Unfortunately, it was time to throw out the first pitch. "Get ready," I told Salty, as he jogged off toward home plate. That was another reason I'd chosen him. As the catcher, it was his job to make pitches look good. And I wanted all the help I could get.

I didn't need it, though. As soon as they introduced us, the crowd was on their feet. It was loud, and as Carlos rolled me to the middle of the infield, it kept getting louder. I pointed at Carlos, *that's my guy*, and the stadium erupted. It was like a full count with the bases loaded. I counted down with my left hand, "Three, two, one," and we threw. Carlos wasn't close. He was three feet outside. It didn't help that Papi dropped the ball.

Salty barely had to move his glove. I painted the corner.

On the video, you can see me yell, "Strike!" with a big smile on my face. My favorite part, though, is the television announcer, who's just talking and then, "Whoa, nice pitch by Jeff Bauman. From the wheelchair." He seems genuinely surprised.

Afterward, we headed toward the EMC level, where the Sox had a section reserved for us. There were a lot of people talking to me, yelling "Boston Strong" and "We're with you, Jeff." Big D was pushing me in my wheelchair, so that I could shake as many hands as I could, and somehow we got lost. We were in a crowd, and we thought we were heading toward a ramp to the EMC level, but it turned out we were being funneled onto an escalator. Suddenly, we were swallowed up, and everyone was pushing forward, and there was no room to double back. When we tried to move to the side, the whole process jammed. Fans ten people behind us were screaming "Come on," and "What's going on up there?"

This was my nightmare: the invalid on the escalator. But before I could say anything, Tim and Big D lifted my wheelchair and stepped onto the escalator, holding me between them. I could hear the yelling slow as people realized what the problem was, and I think I heard someone in the crowd say, "That's Jeff Bauman," but I'm not sure, because I wheeled away as fast as I could as soon as we reached the top.

I spent the rest of the game between my best buds, Carlos and Erin, with a beer in my hand. It seemed like a hundred photos were taken; everyone wanted a photo. We had rounds of food, and rounds of drinks, and eventually my friend Blair—the guy I'd been going to concerts with at the bars in Lowell—was cut off by the bartender for being too drunk, and we all had to let him have some of ours or he wouldn't stop complaining.

After the game, we headed down to the players' parking lot, where a car was waiting for us. I was almost to the car, when I heard "Hey! My friend! Wait up!"

It was Pedro. He said he wanted a photo, so Carlos and I squeezed in with him for a snapshot. Then my friend Blair tried to squeeze in, too.

"I think he's had too much beer." Pedro laughed.

We chatted for almost thirty minutes, while fans in the decks above yelled down at us. Pedro talked with Big D and Tim and everyone, even Blair. When we got in the car, Pedro got in, too, like he was coming home with us.

"All right, Pedro," I said, "let's hit the town."

He laughed and clasped my hand. We did some sort of modified bro shake. "It was great to meet you, my friend," he said.

Hey, Pedro, man, you don't know how great it was. You don't even know.

25.

The next morning, I received my legs. There's part of me that wishes this book was more like a movie, or the video game *Battlefield 4*. I wish this scene was a close-up of a bulletproof vest being put on, and the strap pulled tight. Then the extra ammo clips, the serrated knife, the flash grenades. We see two hands pick up a big gun and lock in a clip, then the camera pulls back and we see two eyes, the only white staring out from a camouflage-painted face, and it's like, *You bombed us, mother-fuckers, now it's our turn.*

I don't want that for the real world. I don't want anyone being bombed or the SWAT team kicking down any doors. That would mean some kid, in some other part of the world, would lose her legs, too, and she wouldn't have the advantages I have. She'd probably never walk again.

But it's like that movie *8 Mile.* It ends with Eminem going back to work...at a factory! Wouldn't it have been better with a ninth mile, one that involved hacking up zombies with a chain saw?

Now *that* would be a good story.

Instead, here's how the story really went down: I sat in a wheelchair, in a small examination room, in a nondescript building in Dorchester. I lifted my leg, put a sock on the end, and unrolled it to the top of my thigh. Then I put on the liner, a thin fabric designed to grip the socket, and unrolled it the same way.

I picked up my artificial leg. I put the socket, a large, thigh-shaped piece of plastic, onto the end of my leg. It wasn't camouflage or black. Maybe those were options, but I'd chosen tie-dye. I shifted my weight, pulling the socket up my thigh, working carefully so that my flesh wouldn't pinch. The fit was tight, but it had to be. Any free space would diminish my strength and could lead to injuries. So I made sure to pull firmly, working the top edge up to my undercarriage, until I felt the raw tip of my leg touching the bottom of the socket. I tightened it once more. Then I grabbed the Velcro near the bottom, pulled it tight, and strapped it along the side of the socket. I guess, if I think hard enough, it was a similar motion to fitting a bullet and locking a rifle, but it didn't feel like that.

I had imagined the moment being like in *Elysium*, when Matt Damon has all the metal parts, and he's kind of bionic. But I didn't feel like Matt Damon. I felt like a gimp.

Mr. Martino checked the legs. I'm not sure what he was doing exactly, but there were screws to turn and electronics to adjust. After a while, I rolled out of the exam room to a hallway with a bar along each wall. I grabbed the bars, and Mr. Martino and his assistants helped me to a standing position.

Wow, what a feeling, to be standing. I felt tall. I had been seeing the world from little-kid height for months; now I felt like an adult again. I felt solid. That's what I remember: I felt solid on my legs. It was an ideal condition. The technicians had helped me to the upright position. I had bars to hold on to. I had people with their hands on my hips in case I slipped. But that didn't take away from the power of that moment. I hadn't expected to feel so good.

"Any pain?" Mr. Martino asked. He was crouched down behind me, examining my legs.

"A little at the bottom."

He adjusted. "How about now?"

"It's pinching."

"That will happen." Another adjustment. "You'll get used to it. The liner should protect you. Does it rub your thigh?"

"Is it supposed to?"

My legs hurt. There was no denying that. But it was a persistent pain, the kind I had learned to live with over the past six weeks. I looked down at my feet. The metal disappeared into a pair of brand-new black Nikes.

I looked up. I could see my reflection in the mirror. I could see the legs extending down from my shorts. The thighs looked huge, but my lower legs were so thin. I was holding myself up with my arms, and I looked strong. Really strong.

"How does that feel?" Mr. Martino asked. He was behind me, making another adjustment.

"I feel good," I said.

I let go of the bars, just for a moment. I was solid.

"Did you see that?" I asked Erin, craning to see behind me.

"See what?"

I lifted my hands again.

"No! Be careful."

I put my hands down on the bars. Erin must have stepped behind me, because I felt her arms around my waist, and then her cheek on my neck. She kissed me. "Does it hurt?"

"No. Not at all."

Mom pulled out her camera. Erin stepped back, and I slowly positioned myself over my thighs until I felt the weight line up, and I was in control. I looked up, smiled, and slowly lifted my hands until they were as high as my shoulders. Mom snapped a photo.

I put my hands back down and then, without really thinking about it ahead of time, I took a step with my right foot. I could hear people gasp.

"Jeff..."

I shifted my left foot and swung it slowly in front. I was staring down at my feet, concentrating. I swung my right foot in front, stopped, and caught my breath. I felt sweat running down my face. My whole back was wet. These steps were taking more effort than I realized. But I wasn't going to quit. I set myself, shifted my weight, and stepped again. Then I looked up, saw Erin, and smiled.

Mom keeps the photograph from that day on the refrigerator at home. It's her favorite picture of me, because it's a picture of triumph. She made three thousand postcards out of it, and she sends them to people who write or send me gifts. Greetings from Boston, Mass., it says right there on the front of my T-shirt.

Thank you, Mom writes on the back.

26.

Boston had turned out for the marathon bombing victims. People had created slogans and wristbands; they had started websites and Facebook pages. The outpouring of support from around the world was so generous, and so many people had started fund-raising efforts, that the state of Massachusetts and the city of Boston created a charity, the One Fund, to organize the contributions. The money raised would be shared among the victims of the bombing based on the severity of our injuries. The primary fund-raising event was a "Boston Strong" concert on May 30—the day after I received my legs—featuring some of the biggest bands in Boston history: Aerosmith, J. Geils Band, New Kids on the Block.

James Taylor, who lived in Brookline, was one of the headliners, and he had invited me to his night-before-the-show rehearsal. It was scheduled for the TD Garden, but the Bruins were making a run to the Stanley Cup finals, and the building was booked. So after I was finished working on my legs (I left them at United Prosthetics for two more days for final adjustments), Kevin picked up Erin and me and took us to the House of Blues, across the street from Fenway, where James Taylor and his band were setting up.

I didn't realize it, but the invitation was the result of weeks of work. Within an hour of our conversation about James Taylor during my first week in the hospital, Kevin had called the media buyers at Costco headquarters in Seattle, Pennie Clark Ianniciello, Stacy Thrailkill, and Judith Logan, who had worked with James Taylor's record label in the past.

"Do you think James could drop by and say hi to Jeff?" he asked them. "It would be a real pick-me-up for him and his girlfriend."

Within twenty-four hours, James Taylor's assistant, Ellyn Kusmin, called Kevin. Mr. and Mrs. Taylor had been following the story; they would be honored to meet me. Kevin worked for weeks to try to coordinate a visit, but it was always a zoo at the hospital, and there wasn't going to be a good time for a quiet visit. Then the concert was organized, and Ellyn told Kevin that James Taylor had "bigger plans than just a hospital visit."

If I had known that part of the story, I would have been more excited. I probably should have been more excited, anyway, even without the details. Instead, I grumbled all the way to the House of Blues. More than once, I tried to back out.

I was crushed. Absolutely exhausted. The Red Sox game was my biggest outing since the bombing, and it had worn me out. Then I had received my legs, and stood for half an hour, and walked those four steps.

I know that doesn't sound like much. I sat in a wheelchair talking with strangers. I threw one pitch, *while sitting down*. I walked four steps. Four!

I know it seems easy. People see me smiling and shaking hands, and they think, it's not so bad, what Jeff has been through. He seems to enjoy it. I've never seen him sad.

It's not like that. Not at all.

I'm not saying I'm faking it. I'm not. I love seeing the people of Boston, and knowing I'm giving back makes it worth it to be alive. But it takes me hours to get up for an event. There is always crushing doubt. I get depressed. Usually, when I arrive, I feel overwhelmed. I don't want to get out of the car. Erin or Big D has to talk me into it. Afterward, when the high of the event has passed, I'm so wiped out, physically and emotionally, that I just want to curl into a ball.

First the Red Sox game. Then United Prosthetics, especially United Prosthetics. It was only four steps, I know, but I don't think I've ever been that tired. The last thing I wanted was to spend another evening in a crowd, shaking hands and smiling.

Then I got to the House of Blues and it was . . . empty. They have an enormous space, and there was almost no one there but a sound guy at his board, and James Taylor's band noodling with their instruments onstage.

Ellyn, James Taylor's assistant, met us at the door. She set Erin and me up in the middle of the room, right in front of the board, where the sound was best. The sound guy came over, and we talked for a minute, and then James Taylor came out and started to play. It was difficult to hear clearly at first, because of the holes in my eardrums. The sound echoed in the empty room, and I couldn't sort out even James Taylor's mellow notes from the distortions and clanging.

And then he played the opening chords of "You've Got a Friend," and the notes started to make sense with one another, and the echoes started to fade. For the rest of the set, it was just me and Erin, alone in front of the soundboard, with James Taylor singing directly to us. I put my arm around her. She put her head on my shoulder, and I thought of our kids, running around in the future on Popsicle stick legs. This was our first date since the bombing.

After the set, James Taylor came down to sit with us. He chatted with Erin, and then she moved off, and it was just him and me. We talked about my first pitch at the Red Sox game, and about receiving my legs. He asked about my future plans, but I told him I didn't have any, I was just focusing on walking for now.

He told me about his life, about not making it in New York and then moving to London, where he auditioned for George Harrison and Paul McCartney, who were thinking about signing him to their record label.

"I hear you're a guitar player," he said.

"I can play a few chords."

He went to the stage and came back with one of his guitars, a Yamaha Acoustic. It was the same guitar I had bought for myself that Christmas, only six months ago, but it felt like a lifetime ago now.

I was worried. I thought he was going to ask me to play with him, and the way my ears were buzzing, I wasn't going to be able to hear the notes.

Instead, he pulled out a marker and wrote on it: *Jeff: Carry on… James Taylor.*

"Thanks," I said, as he handed me the guitar. We talked about playing on the porch on a nice summer day, and about how fun it was to jam with our brothers. James's brother Livingston taught at the Berklee College of Music in Boston and was a sick guitarist himself.

He asked about my medical expenses. I told him I had good insurance, but beyond that I didn't know, nobody had shown me any bills. Mom was taking care of that for me, through an irrevocable trust Uncle Bob had helped set up in my name. Nobody could get money from the trust, even me, without clearing it with the executors.

"I bet you get a lot of donations," he said.

I looked at the ground. The topic made me uncomfortable. "Yeah, I get a lot," I said. "I'm getting money all the time." I rubbed my thighs, my new nervous habit. "I guess I'm going to need it."

"Don't feel bad about it, Jeff," he said. "Just sit back and let people help you. It makes them feel good."

I didn't understand. I still don't understand, not really.

"Yes, sir," I said.

James Taylor laughed. "No need to call me sir."

He invited me to the sound check at the TD Garden the next morning. I asked if I could bring Mom. He said sure, but Mom backed out at the last minute, and Erin had to work, so only Kevin and I got to hear the bands warming up. Musicians and crew kept coming over to us, saying hello, and chatting. Carole King joined James Taylor onstage for "You've Got a Friend." When they got to the chorus, James Taylor smiled and pointed at Kevin and me.

"I guess this will have to be our song," Kevin said.

I laughed. "Sure, Kevy," I said. "Sure."

After his set, James Taylor came over again. He pulled up a chair to sit beside me. He was walking with a cane—maybe he'd had some surgery, I'm not sure. We chatted for a minute, and then someone said loudly, "Move over, James." James Taylor started to move over, but the chairs were spring-loaded, like in a movie theater, and something happened, and before I knew it, he was down on the floor.

"James," the guy yelled, taking his seat. "What happened, James! What are you doing down there?"

It was Jimmy Buffett.

He helped James Taylor back into his chair, made sure he was all right, and then turned back to me. "Can you believe I'm missing fishing in the Bahamas for this?" he said with a smile.

I could see it then: two personalities. Two guys trying to be there for me, each in his own way. They were just different. James Taylor... he was like having a dad. One who comes home after work, takes an interest, asks how you've been.

Jimmy Buffett was like my uncle Bob.

I don't remember much about the concert. They gave about a hundred bombing victims chairs in front of the barriers, so we had in-front-of-the-front-row seats. Erin and both of our moms sat with me. We were too close to the speakers for my ears, so I spent much of the show watching musicians blast away into a sonic fog. After the concert, we went backstage. We met some of the performers, who were generous with their time. We laughed and chatted, and then James Taylor invited my family back to his dressing room, where we hung out for another half hour or so.

By the time I left, the arena was empty, and even Erin and Mom had gone back to the hotel. The Colonnade Hotel, one of the nicest in Boston, had given us free rooms for the night so we wouldn't have to travel back to Chelmsford. Kevin offered to drive me over, so we ended up down in the bowels of the arena with the roadies and Teamsters, winding through passageways, trying to figure out how to get to his car.

Eventually, we passed this heavy dude hanging out by the loading dock. He looked like Silent Bob from the Kevin Smith movies: black clothes, long hair, hat turned backward. "Hey, Jeff, how's it going, man?"

"Good," I said, stopping to shake his hand. I tried to shake everyone's hand I could.

"Did you really see the bomber?" he said.

"I did."

"Really?"

"Yeah. I looked right at him."

"Well, I was reading on the Internet, and there are a lot of inconsistencies in the story. There are a lot of things that just don't make sense..."

"We're out of here," Kevin said. He grabbed my wheelchair and started wheeling me quickly through the tunnels.

The guy ran after us, talking about how the bombing was fake, how it was all a government plot.

Kevin was pissed. He's a nice guy; this was the first time I'd seen him ready to punch somebody in the face. Eventually, the guy stopped following us, and we made it to the car. But Kevin couldn't stop thinking about it. I don't think he said two words on the drive.

Kevin was protective of me. Maybe too protective. He was unhappy with the AP photo of me in the wheelchair. He thought it was an invasion of my privacy, although he later admitted, "It turned out to be a good thing. It gave you the opportunity to prove that wasn't the end of your story."

He thought the conspiracy theories were insulting. That they diminished me and my suffering. I can see that. I got blown up. I lost my legs. I've gone through hell, and so has my family. When people say it's fake, they dismiss our pain. They dump on everything we've done to stick together and find joy in life.

It doesn't bother me, though. Why should it? I understand there is a group of people who think I am an actor, born without legs. That I'm a fake victim of a fake bombing. Why would I do that? I'm not sure. I don't know if they think every victim is a fake, or if all the spectators on that block were fake, or if they think the marathon itself was fake.

I don't want to know. Worrying about conspiracy theories would be like hating the bombers, or obsessively thinking about how things could have gone differently. I don't have time for it. I need my strength. I need to look forward. I can't waste my energy on losers.

As James Taylor sang at the concert, and he pointed right at me when he sang it: "They'll take your soul if you let them, ah, but don't you let them."

The funny thing is, I'm sympathetic to their thinking, at least a bit. The government can't be trusted. They lied about nuclear weapons in Iraq. They kidnap people. They eavesdrop on our conversations. We know these for facts. They even lied about the eavesdropping, on national television, at the exact moment they were doing it to millions of people. They are too big to be punished, and there's nothing we can do about it.

But fake a bombing? At a famous, crowded public event? In a major city in the middle of the day, with thousands of cameras around?

That's stupid.

And it hurts people. It really does. I'm not on the Internet, so I'm not too affected by it, but the reason I'm not on the Internet is because of the conspiracies. (If you Google my name, the first choice is "Jeff Bauman fake.") I don't answer my phone for numbers I don't know, and I keep my voice mail full so strangers can't leave messages. Erin shut down her Facebook page because she didn't want to read the messages.

She has said, at least twice, that she hates the conspiracy theorists more than the bombers.

"The bombers didn't target us," Erin says. "You just happened to be there. But the conspiracy people are trying to ruin our lives. They are terrorizing us, for no purpose, for some stupid hobby."

She doesn't mean it—at least not the part about the "truthers" being worse than the bombers. There's so much anger and frustration, no matter how much we try to stay positive. It comes out in unexpected ways.

It's hardest, I think, for Aunt Jenn. She runs my Facebook page, along with several volunteers, all strangers. She also moderates it, so she hears from the conspiracy nuts. People say terrible things about her and about me. They aren't just dismissing our pain and suffering; they hate us because they think we're government operatives. I tell her to ignore the accusations and threats, but she gets emotional. For a while, she had to stop updating the page, because one person was aggressively attacking her, insisting she talk with him. She couldn't sleep, and she felt unsafe.

"Our family has suffered so much," she said. "Why are they doing this?"

I laughed. "Saying that is just going to make them hate you more, Aunt Jenn."

I have no doubt writing this book will feed the conspiracy. There are all kinds of hidden messages in here, right? Of course! Once someone believes something like that, there's no convincing them otherwise.

It's almost funny.

Except for one thing: Tamerlan Tsarnaev was inspired by conspiracy theories. He believed that 9/11 was an American government plot to frame Muslims, and that lie was so central to his life that he reportedly convinced his own mother it was true. I don't know if the conspiracy started him down the path to murderous hate, or if it was simply a key step in his decline. I think he was a sociopath looking for a reason. But even if 9/11 "truthing" was just an excuse, it wasn't harmless. It was poison.

———————

The day after the concert, Aunt Jenn threw her annual summer party in her big backyard. She lives along a major road in an older house that her husband, Uncle Dale, had owned for decades. A new suburban neighborhood had been built behind it, but their property was grandfathered, so Dale can still park his dump trucks in the back. The yard is so big, you can barely see the trucks behind the pool.

Aunt Jenn usually invited about eighty people to her party, but this year more than 150 came. Instead of the traditional barbecue, she had it professionally catered, and there was a raffle and silent auction. A dozen of my coworkers at Costco came and drank most of the beer. Carlos and Mel were there, along with Kevin. They were all part of our family now.

Two men were jogging from Washington, D.C., to raise money for Martin's family and me. They started at the Pentagon, stopped at Ground Zero, and planned to finish by running the course of the Boston Marathon. I'm not sure where the money came from—I imagine them running along pulling dollars out of bushes, although that's probably not how it worked—but it was an impressive feat. They were scheduled to finish that morning, so Erin ran with them the last ten miles, sprinting down Boylston Street and across the marathon finish line for the first time.

Afterward, the men came to Aunt Jenn's party and gave me a check. Erin gave them her medal for finishing the Boston Marathon. The organizers had given everyone a medal, even those who couldn't finish because of the bombing.

"Don't worry," Erin told the men when they protested. "I'll get a real one next year."

The men left soon after, either because they were tired from their run or because of my shirtless shenanigans, I'm not sure. I was feeling good, riding around in my wheelchair bare-chested, laughing and joking with everyone.

Aunt Jenn kept trying to get me to put my shirt on. She said the sun would turn the burn scars on my torso red. But guess what? Aunt Jenn isn't a doctor. I'm pretty sure she had no idea what she was talking about.

By the time the beer started to run low, though, I was tired. It had been a busy week. But I was happy to be home, and happy to be with my family.

I got out of my wheelchair, sat on the bottom step to Aunt Jenn's aboveground pool, and hauled myself up with my arms. I sat on the edge for a while, enjoying the sunshine and laughing with Erin. Then I flipped myself over into the water.

Aunt Jenn had bought Styrofoam noodles, in case I had trouble staying afloat. I didn't need them. I just spread my arms and floated, weightless and happy, staring at the sky.

27.

On Tuesday, it was back to the grind at Spaulding. Now that I had my prosthetic legs, my workouts changed. I still did the crunches and stretches without my legs, and whatever those exercises are called where you lift your knee (or in my case, thigh) across your body toward the opposite shoulder.

Then I would strap on my Geniums and try the same exercises. Suddenly, what had become natural turned into some real Navy SEAL–type shit. I thought the workouts were hard before, but they were nothing compared to working out with my artificial legs. I lay down on my back and tried to hold my legs off the floor. I lay on my stomach and tried the Superman, lifting my arms and legs straight out at the same time. The first time I did leg presses, it felt like the sockets were going to rip right off my thighs.

Then we'd work on the practical stuff, like standing up from and sitting down in my wheelchair. Michelle put a harness under my crotch with a cord that attached to the ceiling and made me walk between two parallel bars. I hated that; I don't feel comfortable with anything in the undercarriage region. So she switched to a belt, and held on to me from behind while I walked.

The rest of the exercises hurt, but walking was the hardest. Walking involved mental work. I had to concentrate on shifting my weight so I could lift a leg. Then push it forward. Then put it down a few inches in front. I'd stop, focus, then lift the other leg. Nothing was easy. Every step took mental and physical effort. Every shift in my weight took trust that the leg would hold. I'd be huffing after two steps. By the end my shoulders and arms would be sore, because I'd been straining to hold myself up without even knowing it. It took me a full minute to walk ten feet.

Part of it was the Genium legs. They were built with so many fail-safes to stop you from falling that any unorthodox motion locked them out. In the past, you'd see people with artificial legs jutting their hips, then swinging their legs in a half circle, producing a side-to-side swaying walk. This technique took less effort with each step, but cumulatively wore the body down. With the Genium, I had to step correctly each time. The leg wouldn't allow anything else. There were no half measures. No shortcuts. The legs forced me to swap today's pain for tomorrow's gain, and all the other cliches of self-improvement culture. Walking was the most tiring part of my day.

After walking practice, I'd lie on my back for my bridge. In a bridge you lift your torso, hips, and thighs so only your shoulders and feet are touching the ground. Most of the upward force comes from the legs, but it's the thighs and core that hold the position. My legs, though, couldn't produce upward force, because they were inanimate metal rods. And I struggled to keep my feet from slipping. Bridging meant controlling my weight while exerting maximum force and stretching my torso in a backward arch. It combined balance, strength, and flexibility.

"The bridge is the key," Michelle told me every session. "Once you can do a one-legged bridge on each side, you'll have all the strength and coordination you need."

It was so important, she wouldn't consider moving on to more complicated processes, like walking on slanted surfaces or stairs, until I mastered it. Until I could hold my two-legged bridge for thirty seconds, I was stuck with small steps on the parallel bars.

I could handle the physical exertion. I was used to it by then, and I'd seen progress. I was obviously stronger, if not necessarily confident. It was the rest of my life that was becoming a struggle. Erin was working five days a week, and the effort was wearing her down. Her boss was understanding, letting her take an occasional morning off to spend with me at Spaulding, or an extralong lunch so we could relax in Boston after my workout. They let her switch her schedule so that she could leave at three to beat the traffic back to Chelmsford.

It didn't work. Even leaving at three, it took her two hours to get to Mom's apartment. By then, she was worn out and cranky, and I was anxious. The joy of being alone in my room had turned into loneliness. My body needed rest, but I couldn't sleep, so the days crept by. Mom was trying; she was working hard to give me what I needed, but I didn't want to . . . hang out with her. And since I couldn't drive, I was trapped in the apartment. It was a mile to any business besides a bank, with no sidewalk.

I had visitors, but I was beginning to lose patience with some of the people who came by. Aunt Jenn, for instance, was always trying to get me to open up about my feelings. Several articles had quoted me as saying that after the explosion, I thought I was going to die, and that I was okay with that.

"I want to talk about it," Aunt Jenn told me. "I'm not comfortable with that feeling."

I didn't want to talk about it. Unless you've been there, how can you understand? I looked down that day, and my legs were applesauce.

I saw my feet, and they weren't attached to my body.

Maybe it would be better if I didn't remember that so clearly, because once you've seen something like that, you don't sleep. I'm not sure I'll ever sleep well again.

I didn't want to die. No way. I wanted to live. But my body had been ripped apart; I was lying in a pool of my own blood, and when that happens, you die. There was nothing I could do about it. I was going to die. So I accepted it. I saw the good in my life. I was happy for the time I had.

Maybe that doesn't make me a fighter. Maybe even though acceptance lasted only a second, until Carlos Arredondo lifted me up, that doesn't gibe with the "no pain, no gain, work hard, play hard, never give up" style of looking at the world. Maybe a true hero would have screamed, *Hell no.*

But I'm not that guy.

"Okay, I understand," Aunt Jenn said when I didn't respond. "You're not ready. I understand. But one day, Jeff, we're going to talk about everything."

No we're not, Aunt Jenn. I'm not *that* guy, either.

I preferred Derek and Sully, who never asked me anything. I bought a flat-screen television, put it in my room, and we'd play PlayStation. *EA Sports. MLB: The Show.*

I preferred the Red Sox, who were slowly pulling away from the rest of their division, despite their lack of stars.

But Derek and Sully both worked: Derek for Uncle Bob, and Sully for his stepfather (who was divorced from his mother, but broken family is still family). Derek often came by in the afternoon, when Uncle Bob gave him time off to hang with me. Sully would disappear for days.

So I spent most of the afternoon alone. Playing video games. Fiddling with my guitar. I'd break out my orange amps (another gift) and play my olive-colored Epiphone, the one the guy in Oregon had given me, until my damaged ears were ringing. It helped me forget what the days were really like. How my life was going to be. I'd learn to drive one day. I'd learn to walk. But I'd always be limited in what I could do.

I could never play pickup basketball. Never join a coed softball team. Never run. Never fly a plane.

I couldn't go back to my old job at Costco, carrying heavy loads of food to the displays, turning rotisserie chickens, standing at a counter chopping vegetables. And the last thing I wanted was to be given a handicapped job. I didn't want to be some sort of greeter, like a store mascot. If I was at the front of the store, with my artificial legs, it would be a circus.

I wanted Erin. She didn't have to ask what I needed, because she knew what I was going through. She would tell me to lie down when she knew my legs were hurting. She would give me a hug when I woke up in the morning and tried to get out of bed. I had terrible nightmares. I don't remember what they were about, but I'd wake up sweating and feverish. Erin would rub my back, sometimes for an hour, until I calmed down enough to lie still.

"Move in with me," I'd tell her.

She'd sigh. "I can't do that."

She was practically living out of her car. She was staying with me at Mom's four or five nights a week, but there wasn't room for her stuff. She had her clothes in the backseat, hauling them back and forth between Boston and Chelmsford. When she wasn't with me, she'd stay at her apartment in Brighton, or she'd drive to her parents' house and stay the night with them. Remy and Michele had gone home for the summer to recover from their wounds, so I think her parents' house was the only place she felt comfortable.

"Move in with me," I'd tell her.

And she'd say, "Not here, Jeff. I can't move in here."

I needed her. Without Erin, my life was hell. I was lonely. I couldn't sleep. I'd lie awake thinking about the bombing, feeling depressed and tense for hours. It wasn't sights or sounds, or even smells, that troubled me. It was the feeling of helplessness. Of lying in the street with no legs and no way to get up. There were nights on end when I never slept at all, not for a second.

Most days, I'd start texting Erin after lunch.

What time u comin?

Don't know. Tired today. Maybe I'll stay at apartment.

I need you. About 6?

I'm tired, Jeff.

My legs hurt.

No response.

I'll take you to dinner.

No response.

I love you.

OK.

28.

Despite my new legs and lack of sleep, I stayed busy in June. I went to my friend's bachelor party at a gun range. Erin's sister Gail drove us to Rhode Island for a toddler cousin's birthday party, the first time I met her extended family. Then Erin and I went to New Jersey to spend time with my dad's family, who threw a party and fund-raiser in my honor. A company called Now City gave me a free helicopter ride over Boston.

There was a poker tournament to raise funds for Pitching In for Kids, a charity that raised money to pay for children's hospital bills supported by Red Sox legends Tim Wakefield and Jason Varitek. I blew the starter horn for the Falmouth Seven Mile on Cape Cod, then waited for Erin at the finish line with a sign that said, "Go Erin. Run Like a Girl." I spoke to a class at Boston University's medical school. I recorded a public service announcement for the Boston Athletic Association, the sponsors of the marathon, supporting and thanking emergency responders.

At every event, strangers would come up to me. They would shake my hand or want pictures. "Sure, what's your name?" Women, from grandmothers to teens, would ask if they could give me a hug. "Of course." Kids would ask for my autograph. "Do you want me to write it on your hand, or that napkin?"

I tried not to turn anyone down, even the people who wanted to tell me where they were on the day of the bombing, what they saw, how they felt when they saw the picture of me. I don't like to talk about the bombing. I'd rather talk about anything else.

Kat, who was used to helping with crowds, often went with me. And I always had at least one of my crew—Sully, Big D, or my brother

Tim—and not just because I needed a ride. I didn't feel safe without them. I didn't like looking around and realizing I didn't recognize anyone. And my boys were fun, too. They were the perfect companions for the VIP section, where the booze was free.

The other person with me at every event was Carlos, because the organizers always invited us together. He was always smiling, always wearing his famous cowboy hat. Early on, he had given me a cowboy hat just like his, but I never wear it. I keep it in a special spot in my room. Carlos wasn't a drinker; he was a talker. He was a "Dad on Fire" with a simple message: love the troops enough to stop the wars. Many times, I would be chatting with Carlos when he'd suddenly disappear. I always knew where I'd find him: with soldiers. Carlos talks with every soldier he sees, especially Marines. His son Alex was a Marine.

Erin was more than happy to miss these events. People always asked for her, because she was well-known in Boston, but she didn't like the attention. When she ran the last ten miles with the two men from Washington, D.C., she tried to run away from the reporters. She was often recognized on the street. Not as much as me, because . . . you know, the legs. If someone thought they recognized me, all they had to do was check what was going on below the waist. If you were in your twenties in Boston that summer, with dark hair and no legs, I bet it sucked. You'd keep being mistaken for Bauman.

Erin enjoyed the nights off when I went to charity events. Her life with me was stressful. The longer she stayed with me, the more she took over the tasks Mom had originally handled. She was my driver, errand runner, and reacher for things on the top shelf of the refrigerator. She emptied my pee cup.

"Erin," I'd call, "I have a present for you."

"Oh great," she'd joke. "Still warm."

She never got much sleep. I tossed and turned too violently in bed. I often suffered terrible cramping at night, probably because of anxiety, so Erin would wake up at two or three in the morning and massage my legs. My rubbings, we called them. But no happy endings. I was too sore, and my God, I ran hot. While Erin was rubbing out my tension, I was sweating like a monkey.

She also handled my schedule and worked with Kat on media requests.

"I'm not your social secretary," she would say with exasperation when another publicist called her to see if I could make an appearance. "Why can't you handle this?"

"Just tell them no."

"It's a charity, Jeff. For kids with cancer."

"Tell them yes. I'll definitely do that. When is it?"

"I have a full-time job, you know."

"And I don't have any legs."

I'd smile when I said stuff like that. I didn't mean it.

Erin's mom, Lori, finally called me. I love Erin's parents. They are the most low-key people I've ever been around. They were so respectful of our space that on the first Saturday I was in the hospital, almost a week after the bombing, I had to ask where they were. I was disappointed they hadn't visited me.

"They've been here the whole time," someone said. They had stayed mostly in the family area, making sure that Erin and everyone else, even strangers, had the support they needed. They knew my family was a circus. They hadn't wanted to intrude on my time.

"Send them in," I said immediately. "I want to see them."

They had been like that throughout my recovery. Erin's mom called her every Wednesday, to offer support, but she never pressured her. That's why Erin usually went home when I had a charity event, because her parents gave her the space to relax. She needed to sleep, to exercise, to eat a home-cooked meal. She probably needed time away from her "mother-in-law." Mom loved Erin, but it's tough for your girlfriend to spend so much time in your mom's five-hundred-square-foot apartment.

Erin and her mom often talked for hours, I knew, when Erin went home. They were very close. So I listened when Lori called. This was the first time she'd reached out to me directly, so I knew it was important.

Erin was stressed, Lori told me. I was putting too much pressure on her. Erin wanted to be there for me, because she loved me and she knew I needed it, but she needed to take care of herself, too.

She was exhausted. When she was home, she cried. A lot. She had so much guilt and anger. There were so many feelings pulling her in so many different directions that she didn't know what to do. She felt like her life was out of control.

"I know you've been through a lot," her mom said. "I'm not saying you're doing anything wrong. It's just . . . Bill and I are here for you, Jeff. If you need anything, please call us. We will do whatever you need."

"Move in with me," I said that night, when Erin and I were lying in my bed together. It was a one-person bed. Neither one of us ever got much sleep.

"I can't move in here, Jeff. It will only work if we have our own place."

I had received my payout from the One Fund. It was the highest level, since my injuries were in the most severe category, and it was a large amount of money. Along with the money sent to my Facebook page, and other fund-raisers like the event at the Chelmsford Radisson, I had been given . . .

Well, I don't want to say how much exactly. Let's just say that at my old salary, I would have had to work at Costco for almost exactly two hundred years to make that much.

Thanks to Uncle Bob, the money was safely put away in a trust. It was conservatively invested, and beyond regularly scheduled payouts, I wasn't allowed to touch it. If I wanted something larger, like a house, the trustees had to approve the expense.

That was the best way to assure the money would be used as

intended—for my medical treatments and basic needs—and would last my whole life. I wasn't worried that I'd buy anything extravagant. I'm not interested in that. But I might have been tempted to buy PlayStations for all those kids with "Bauman Strong" lemonade stands.

"Let's get a small apartment," Erin said. "In the city, on the ground floor, close to my office."

"I don't know."

"Let's get a dog. Let's cook dinner at home and see how it goes."

I had told Erin moving in with Mom was only temporary, a few weeks at most. It had already been a month, but the longer I stayed, the harder it was to imagine moving out.

"Move in with me here," I told her. "It will be so much easier for you."

"No, Jeff," she said, "it won't be easier. Not unless I quit my job, leave my friends in Boston. But I like my life."

"No you don't. You're tired all the time."

"Well...I liked it before."

I kissed her, and she kissed me back. We kissed for a while. "Move in with me," I said. "You're staying here most nights, anyway. What's the worst that could happen?"

Erin didn't say anything for a while. So I rolled over, put my arm around her, and listened to her breathing. She was probably thinking of the worst that could happen, but I have no idea what that might have been. She shared with her mother, but she never really shared with me. Not her deepest anxieties, anyway. I was her patient as well as her love. She didn't feel like she could burden me.

"I don't want to quit my job," she said.

"I can take care of you, Erin. I have money now."

"I know. That's what I'm worried about."

29.

Kevin came by Mom's apartment with a care package from Costco at least once a week. It's strange to have your boss—and not just your boss, but the boss of your boss—show up at your house, but I guess, by then, Kevin was more than my store manager. "Sir" was out. When I called him "Heavy Kevy" now, it was more like the way I called Derek "Big D"—a sign that he was one of us.

He could never remember not to park right in front of Mom's building, though. That killed me. There was an older woman who lived upstairs and stared out her window most of the day, and she'd always yell at him, "Who are you?"

Kevin would have his hands full: maybe a signed poster, or some day-old flowers for Mom, or some food that was too old to be sold in the deli but was still delicious. "I'm Kevin, remember? I'm here to see Jeff."

"Well, you can't park there. That's reserved parking."

"I'm sorry. I'll only be a minute."

Kevin never stopped supporting me, and neither did Costco. I hadn't worked there in more than two months, but I was still part of their family. Kevin told me the regional manager for the Northeast still asked about me—he had visited me at Boston Medical Center—and still passed on information to Pennie, Stacy, Judith, and all the others at headquarters in Seattle.

It was Judith's idea, in fact, to send Will and Byron, two Costco employees from the Seattle area who had also lost legs. The company flew them to Boston and put them up at the Colonnade Hotel for a few days. The Colonnade had donated rooms for the One Fund concert,

172 | JEFF BAUMAN

and Kevin had become friends with the manager. Honestly, give that guy five minutes, and he could become friends with anyone. He and Uncle Bob—who were in many ways opposites—had become such good friends that they had started going to Red Sox games together.

They were even planning a Patriots football trip, too.

So Kevin picked me up in Chelmsford, and we drove to the Colonnade to hang out with his "good friends" Will and Byron, whom he'd met for the first time that morning. I wasn't too sure about this meeting, considering the only thing I had in common with these guys was missing legs, and I didn't really want to talk about being crippled with a couple of cripples. It kind of bugged me, honestly, that someone thought I would.

We met in the hotel lobby, then went to the samurai exhibit at the Museum of Fine Arts. I had been into samurai ever since the woman in Japan had sent me the small ceramic and cloth armor replica. It was a great exhibit, but I cramped up from sitting in my wheelchair so long, so afterward we went to an out-of-the-way lobby where I could lie down and stretch out. Byron can talk about anything with anyone, so for a long time we avoided the subject that was noticeably absent below our thighs.

Finally, Byron said, "What you got for scars?"

"Oh, I've got scars," I said. I lifted my shirt to show him the foot-long surgery scar running down my stomach. It was an ugly red thing.

"I've got the same one," Byron said. He lifted his shirt. Byron had my scar, but he also had eight or nine more, running across his torso.

Byron had been moving a load of lumber in his pickup truck. The load shifted, so he pulled over to the side of the road to adjust it. He had the tailgate down, standing behind his truck, when a driver high on heroin swerved off the road and hit him full speed. The tailgate sliced off both his legs, and the rest of his body went flying through the air and into a ditch. I couldn't believe he was still alive, sitting here talking with me. He had been in a coma for a month.

"I was scheduled to be working that day," Byron said. "I switched with a friend so he could attend his kid's birthday party the next day."

If Byron had been working, no accident. No matter the situation, there's always a what-if.

"That's nothing," Will said, lifting his shirt. Will was missing an ear and had burns on his scalp, but that didn't prepare me for the damage on the rest of his body. He had been asleep on a long car trip when his friend tried to pass on a two-lane country road and rammed into an oncoming car. Four people, including Will's friend, died. Will was thrown through the windshield into the other car, which burst into flames. Let's just say Will is totally badass for walking and talking right now.

"I'm luckier than you," Will said with a laugh. "I still have a leg." Will was only missing one joint. He was below-the-knee on the right side only, but I'm sure it still took him years to consider himself lucky.

"What kind of legs you got?" Byron asked me.

I told him about the Geniums. Byron, a four-joint double amputee like me, had the previous version, the C-Leg. "They will last about five years, maybe seven if you're lucky," he told me. "I have to have mine repaired all the time."

"What do you do, run marathons?" I joked.

"No," he said, "I ride dirt bikes."

Byron lived in a rural area outside Seattle, near Mount Rainier. He had a wife, kids, and a dirt bike track in his back acreage that he'd built himself, with jumps and everything. He pounded his legs over those jumps at forty or fifty miles an hour. He was active as hell.

"I'm coming out there for some jumps," I told Byron.

"Do you ride dirt bikes?" he said.

"It doesn't matter, Byron. I can handle some jumps."

We talked for hours, at the museum and then over dinner. We talked about anger. "I'm not angry," I told them. "I'm just confused."

We talked about pain, and how to manage it. We talked about

frustration. We talked about family, and how hard it was on them, and how much effort went into making those relationships work. Will hadn't been married at the time of the accident, but now he had a wife and five kids. He was working it! I don't know if Will and Byron said it directly, but it was obvious that all the work they had put in was worth it. They had it hard, no doubt, but they loved their lives.

And in the end, that was exactly what I needed to hear. Even my best days were full of depression and worry. Anything could trigger an episode—the sound of a firework, a curb I couldn't get over, a backpack strapped across someone's shoulder. The feelings usually lasted only a few minutes, especially if Erin was there to soothe me, but they were part of my life now.

And more and more, they were forcing me to confront something else: that this was forever. All these slights and frustrations, they were my life now.

I hated that. I hated the way the worry crawled up into my mind at odd times and made me self-conscious, and how it was always there in the background, a weight to carry, trying to crush me down.

I didn't know I had that weight, until Byron and Will helped me carry it. I was inspired by my fellow survivors, because we were in this together. I will never forget the soldiers who visited us at Spaulding, because they made me believe. But Will and Byron were different. They showed me the future. They were ten years down the road, and they were happy. Their lives weren't crippled at all. Their lives were whatever they wanted them to be.

30.

Sometime in this period, as I struggled with the *permanence* of my injuries, Erin quit her job. It was a hard decision for her, because it went against her nature. She had been supporting herself since she was twenty years old.

"I'm not the kind of person who would give up everything for someone else," she confided to Kat.

But she'd already given up so much: her social life, her neighborhood in Boston, her sense of self. When I met Erin, she had known who she was and what she wanted. That was one of the things I loved about her. But now who was she, outside of my caretaker? And how much was she allowed to want?

"I don't want to give up myself," she said. "Not forever. Not even for Jeff."

"You're not," Kat said. "You're a hero in all this, too."

I still remember Erin's words from the hospital: *When I saw you smiling, I knew you were still my person. I knew there was nowhere else I wanted to be.*

But what did being with me mean? And how much did she have to give up?

"It's only temporary," Erin told me. "Until we get everything straightened out. Then I'm going back to work."

"Whatever you need, my magical wonderful. I'm just happy you're here."

It was incredible to have Erin around so much. Nightmares, panic attacks, sudden pain: it was all easier to manage with Erin. She made my life easier in practical ways, too. She helped me with my stretches.

She drove me to Spaulding. She helped me put on and take off my legs. I was using a walker now, instead of the parallel bars, so I could practice at home. I tried to walk an hour a day, around and around the tiny apartment. I needed a flat surface. I couldn't handle grass, or those small pebbles that are always in parking lots. Even the ramp outside Mom's front door threw off my balance because it changed the angle between my lower leg and foot. Erin made sure I worked every day.

"Don't get frustrated," she'd tell me. "You're doing great."

We ordered takeout a lot, since neither of us were comfortable cooking in Mom's kitchen. Sometimes, we ordered takeout three times a day, an admission that still makes Erin almost sick. She was never a fan of takeout, but I found short trips to restaurants even more difficult than longer outings.

The first time Mom and I went to Zesty's, for instance, it was horrible, and not just because it took five minutes to get out of the car. Mom struggled with the wheelchair, and I was still figuring out how to grip the doorframe and lift myself out.

It was horrible because I'd been going to Zesty's forever, and I had known the people there for most of my life. They knew me in sixth grade, when all the kids would come to Mom's apartment complex to play manhunt, because the complex was huge and Mom always let us stay up late. They knew me when I was an expert on every free playground in Chelmsford, and when Sully spun a one-eighty trying to drag race a Saturn down a winding road. One time, Mom took me to Zesty's to buy chicken fingers. Mom didn't have enough money, and her credit card was declined. They gave me the chicken fingers anyway.

"You can pay us later," they told Mom. They didn't have to do that for us, but they did, and that's why I'll never forget it.

And now, after all those years, Zesty's felt different. They were incredibly nice. They all wanted to talk. They wanted to tell me how proud they were of my bravery, my attitude, my helping catch the bombers.

Terrible. Those animals. Boston Strong.

I smiled and laughed, but inside I was dying. It wasn't the same. It was like . . . I wasn't one of them anymore. I was a freak. It was a homecoming, but I just wanted to go home.

Mom didn't understand. She was upset that I hadn't been more social. "They care about you, Jeff." She made me feel guilty. Or maybe I should say more guilty than I already felt.

It wasn't just that everyone was nice; they gave me stuff, too. Free food. Free beer. Restaurants had pictures of me on the walls, alongside their Boston Strong banners. I don't see that as much now, but that summer, when the bombing was fresh, Boston Strong and I were everywhere. The Brickhouse even had a huge framed photo of me throwing the first pitch at the Sox game. It's still there. I love it. It's in the men's bathroom, though, and that makes it awkward. Public bathrooms are tough enough in a wheelchair. It doesn't help when you're staring at yourself from the wall.

Thank God the Hong Kong had three steps outside the front door. I never had to worry about accidently ending up in there.

Erin understood my frustration. "You don't have to do anything you aren't comfortable with," she told me. "You don't owe anyone anything."

She always told me that: *You don't owe anyone, not friends, not the media, not Boston. You need to focus on yourself.*

But I wasn't so sure.

A few days before Erin quit her job, the Boston Bruins had called again. The team had made an unexpected run to the Stanley Cup Finals against the Chicago Blackhawks. It was a best-of-seven series, and the two teams had split the first four games. Win or lose the next one, they would be back in Boston on Monday for a pivotal Game 6.

My last appearance as flag captain had gone well. The crowd loved it. "We got so many e-mails and tweets," the media rep said. "It was the most inspirational flag ceremony we've ever done." The Bruins wanted me to come back and recapture the magic. But with one twist: they wanted me to walk.

Not a chance.

I mean, I was doing pretty well with the walker. I hadn't fallen once. But that had been for only a week, and only at the Spaulding gym and around the apartment. I still had to concentrate on every step. Ten steps still crushed me.

There was no way I could walk out in front of thirty thousand people. No way.

I had to tell the Bruins no, but I felt so badly about it. I felt like I was letting everyone down. This was Game 6! A championship was on the line! Obviously, people thought I could walk. They just *assumed* it. Maybe that's because they knew people who had lost both their legs and walked two months later?

Maybe, I thought, that's because I'm behind.

The Bruins called back. They had changed the plan: now they just wanted me to stand.

That night, Erin, Mom, and I argued. Or more precisely, Erin and Mom argued. Erin said what she always said: that I shouldn't feel pressured to do something I wasn't comfortable with, and that standing in front of a crowd, on television, was clearly *too much*. She was angry, I think, at the Bruins. She felt they were pushing me too hard.

Mom said I had to do it. I was a symbol of hope and courage. I had to do everything I could, not just for the Bruins, but for the city.

I didn't say anything. I just listened. After a while, I rolled myself into my room and picked up my guitar. After a few minutes, Erin came in and sat with me. She rubbed my back.

"It's your decision, Jeff," she said.

Mom must have been upset, because she started drinking. By midnight, she was outside my locked bedroom door, yelling that I couldn't let this opportunity pass, that I had to help while I could. People care now, she said, but it wasn't always going to be this way.

She'd leave for a while, then come back. Sometimes she was crying. Sometimes she was yelling. Sometimes she'd start out talking, then switch to yelling, then end up in tears. "Something special is happening, Jeff. You are inspiring people. How can you turn them down? How can you say no after what everyone has done for you? You owe them.

"This will be over soon," she said. "This attention. But your recovery won't be. It will go on and on. So take the good while you can, Jeff, because the world doesn't give for long."

It went on like that for three hours, until Erin and I were exhausted, and Mom had worn herself out.

"Is it like this often?" Erin asked, when the apartment was finally quiet.

I shrugged. It didn't seem like a big deal. "It's been like this all my life," I said.

She hugged me, although I didn't need it.

"You're right," I said. "We should get our own place."

31.

Actually, both Mom and Erin were right. That was what kept me up all night thinking about the Boston Bruins. That and the pain.

I really did need to take care of myself first. That began with my rehabilitation. I needed to work out harder and longer, with even more focus. The first few steps on my artificial legs had been a revelation, but also a false hope. If I can walk ten feet, I thought, then walking a thousand won't be that hard.

It was harder than I imagined. There were so many things that could go wrong: weakness in my thighs, my upper body being off balance, my leg locking because I stepped on a sloped surface, or, say, a letter that had fallen on the floor. I had given myself a year to learn to walk. To try to walk after only two and a half months, almost ten months before everyone told me it would be possible . . . it wasn't realistic.

I needed to be at peace with that. I needed to accept my limitations. Otherwise, I would always be frustrated. Already, I was frustrated every day by what I couldn't do, by my fear of being in a crowd and my discomfort with people staring at me. It was depressing. When I failed at simple tasks, it made me feel not only different, but less than what I had been.

Did I really need to go in front of thirty thousand people with the sole purpose of standing up, when standing up was so . . . so nothing to them? And when there was a pretty good chance I couldn't do it?

On the other hand, the city of Boston had given me so much. Those thirty thousand people at the hockey game had watched my struggles and supported me. They had sent me gifts. If I was a symbol of hope and courage, like so many people said, didn't I need to embrace that role? Wasn't it my responsibility to be courageous? To stand up for the city when it called on me?

If I really could make people feel better, how could I refuse?

No, it wasn't the city calling. It was only a hockey team. But this was *Boston's* hockey team. And it was the Stanley Cup. How could I pass on a chance to help the Bruins win a championship?

You can make a difference. That's what Mom had said to me. *The way you act, Jeff, makes a difference in people's lives. That's what they are responding to, your kindness and strength. Maybe you didn't ask for this, but it's yours. For now. Show them that no matter what happens in their lives, they can overcome it.*

Show us that we matter. That tragedy can make us strong.

I talked about it with my physical therapist, Michelle, at my workout the next day. I could tell she wasn't for it, and I knew she was right. I wasn't ready.

But was waiting the best option? Wasn't she always saying I needed to push myself?

"If I do it, will you come with me?"

This was a big request. I loved Michelle. A lot of people thought she was a hard-ass, especially when they first met her. And she was. She'd push me past my breaking point, and then she'd turn to the next exercise and say, "Keep going. No breaks." But once you warmed up to her, she was funny. We laughed a lot. She was only trying to help.

But she wasn't my friend. She was someone I paid to spend time with me. And now I was asking her to give me a whole evening, free of charge.

She didn't hesitate. "If you want to do this, Jeff, I'll be there for you."

This time, I was prepared for the quiet and darkness as Carlos rolled me to the middle of the arena. I was prepared for the flashing lights playing across the ice, the booming announcer, and the sea of people that roared around me as the houselights came on. Michelle was beside me, but I didn't need her. I grabbed my walker with two hands and pulled myself to a standing position. Carlos waved the Boston Strong flag as I raised my right hand and waved to the crowd.

They went bah-nanas. They were ready. I had given as much as I could.

The Bruins had offered me a luxury box, but I told them I wanted to sit in the crowd this time. We ended up a few rows back, close enough to hear the rattling of the boards and yell at the Blackhawks. Some Watertown cops happened to be sitting a few seats down from us, including their chief of police, Ed Deveau. These guys were in the late-night shoot-out that killed Tamerlan. They were there when the FBI captured Dzhokhar. We were swapping stories the whole time. They were some of the cops who told me, "Don't ever doubt what you did for the investigation, Jeff. You're a hero." But these guys were the heroes. They risked their lives to capture the bombers. By the third period, we were hugging each other. It was an honor to be in the same story as those guys.

Afterward, Big D pulled his car into the handicap-accessible area outside the arena to pick me up. The Bruins had lost a lead in the final period, surrendering two quick goals, and the Blackhawks had just celebrated a championship on our ice. We were bummed as I swung myself into the car.

"Let's hit it, Big D," I said, strapping up.

Someone knocked on my window. I looked out. A guy in a Bruins jersey was standing there, signaling to me. I rolled down my window.

"Jeff Bauman," he said. I'm pretty sure he was drunk. "I just wanted to shake your hand, bro."

"Thank you," I said, shaking his hand.

As he left, someone else stepped forward. "Great to see you tonight, Jeff."

"Thank you. It's nice to meet you."

Another person stepped forward. Then another one.

"We have to go," Big D said.

"It's cool," I said, shaking another hand. "We got time." I went through five or six more people, some of them talking with me, some of the women kissing me on the cheek. They said I inspired them. I told them they inspired me, too.

"We really need to go, Jeff," Big D said again.

"Chill," I said, "one more minute."

"Dude...it's not going to be one more minute. There's a line down the block."

I looked out the window. There must have been a hundred people waiting to shake my hand, and more were piling into the back of the line.

A few minutes later, we pulled away. I waved to the line as we left, and the whole line waved back. It was one of the most memorable moments of my summer. I hadn't been sure I wanted to be at the game. I was never sure I wanted to go anywhere, honestly. It was always a struggle. Always.

But it always ended the same way: I was so happy I'd come.

A few days later, I sat down for my one national television interview, with Brian Williams of NBC. He had called Kat personally, which impressed me so much I stuck with him, despite a last-minute call from Oprah's people. Mom was devastated. She loved Oprah. But I'd made a promise. I couldn't go back on my word.

That interview was the first time I used the word *stronger*. Mr. Williams asked me, "How are you different from before the marathon?"

"I'm stronger," I replied. "Way stronger."

I meant physically. At Spaulding, they called me Wolverine, after the X-Man, because of the way my wounds healed. I could do a hundred push-ups, no problem, when I had never even attempted that before. I had mastered the one-leg bridge. I was physically strong.

But I was stronger in other ways, too. I just hadn't realized it yet.

32.

We went to Uncle Bob's house on the South Shore of Maine in mid-July. Our family went every summer. It was as much a tradition as Aunt Jenn's barbecue in June and Cole's birthday party in August. Uncle Bob's house was pimped out, and it was right on the beach. I've never been a beach person—so much sand—but it was nice to swim in the ocean on a hot July day.

As it turned out, that was the week of the *Rolling Stone* controversy. The magazine had released an issue with a huge close-up of Dzhokhar Tsarnaev, the younger bomber, on the cover. It was sort of a glamour shot. It wasn't from a photo shoot, but it was a photo that made him look about as handsome and "rock star" as he could ever look.

People were upset, especially in Boston. There had been a protest against the magazine, and a Massachusetts State Police sergeant named Sean Murphy had, without authorization, given photos of the manhunt to *Boston* magazine. The photos showed cops in riot gear, and Dzhokhar covered with blood, trying to exit the boat where he was found. One showed the red dot of a rifle target on his bloody face. This is what the magazine should have published, he said.

That, of course, created its own controversy.

Sergeant Murphy, who had initially been suspended from the force, happened to be at his summer place in the same small Maine town. Uncle Bob's friend Gerry Callahan, the radio personality, said the sergeant wanted to meet me. I said sure, tell him to come by. I met cops all the time. I loved meeting cops.

We had lunch, chatted, and took a picture afterward. Soon after, Aunt Jenn uploaded the photo to Facebook. The next morning, there was a big article in the newspaper, featuring the photo, claiming that I supported Sergeant Murphy. Before long, it was national news. I didn't feel anyone had done anything wrong, but other people started to feel like I was being manipulated. That maybe Mr. Callahan, who was outspoken on the issue, was using me to help Sergeant Murphy.

"I don't want to make a statement," I told Kat, when she advised me to clear up the misperception. "I just want it to go away."

I wasn't against Sergeant Murphy. I don't think he should have released the photos. And I also don't think he should have been reassigned to the graveyard shift, which was what eventually happened. It was an emotional time. Very emotional. We should all have second chances.

I was just worried that everything would get blown out of proportion. And it did. With the photo circulating, the press dug up something I had said on my radio interview with Gerry Callahan on WEEI, a minor controversy at the time. Mr. Callahan asked what I thought of Tamerlan Tsarnaev, and I responded, "He's dead, and I'm still here."

It wasn't meant to be vengeful. I wasn't saying I wanted him dead, or that I was happy he had died. It was a statement of fact. Who came out better because of the bombing? Nobody. But that coward got it worse than me.

Now the press was putting that statement and the photo together, implying that I was offended by the *Rolling Stone* cover, and violently angry toward the Tsarnaev brothers.

This was crazy.

And wrong.

I don't have vengeance in my heart against the bombers. I don't want to see the surviving brother tortured or executed or taken out vigilante style. I don't necessarily want him dead. I don't want him walking free, able to hurt other people, but I don't see how his death accomplishes anything. It's not closure for me. What they did is part of my life, whether the bombers are alive or not.

I respect people who think differently. Aunt Jenn and Mom hate the bombers for what they've put us through. They call them monsters and animals.

"They don't deserve to be on this planet," Aunt Jenn says.

Mom keeps it simple. "They killed people, Jeff," she says. "They killed a child. Martin's parents had to watch their son die. Only a monster would do that."

No, I thought, they were people. No matter what they did, they were people.

I never thought about them beyond that. Why? I don't know. Maybe it's part of my healing. Maybe I'll go through an angry phase one day, like the psychologist at Spaulding said I might. But the people I think about, when it's quiet and I have to think about the bombing, are the Odoms, who were with my family in the hospital; Ms. Corcoran, who lost her legs and almost lost her daughter; Pat and Jess, the newlyweds; Martin, Krystle, and Lingzi Lu, who stood near me, but whom I never got to meet.

I think about Carlos.

All those friends inspire me.

It didn't bother me that *Rolling Stone* wrote about Dzhokhar Tsarnaev. I didn't want to read the article, and I never have, but I wasn't upset that they tried to understand why he would bomb a marathon and kill innocent people. It's important to know, because he wasn't a monster. He was a kid.

I felt kind of bad for him, actually. Not as bad as I did for the victims, but a little. He was only nineteen, and when you're nineteen, you do stupid stuff. I did, and you probably did, too. Sure, very few people do something that stupid or evil—and there's no other word for it; blowing up strangers is evil—but he was still just a depressed teenager acting like a jerk.

You get only two or three important choices in life. What job you do, whom you marry. Those are big decisions. If you're right about those two decisions, you'll probably be happy.

Dzhokhar Tsarnaev made the worst decision possible. He destroyed his own life, and he took out innocent people in the process. He's nineteen, and he won't have a chance to make any other important decisions. He's done.

I don't want to give his defense any ideas. I don't want them to say, "Jeff Bauman isn't angry at my client," because that's not my place. We should decide his fate together, because that's what our country is about. I hope he stays in jail forever.

But still, I mostly blame his brother. Tamerlan Tsarnaev and I, we were similar. We were both twenty-seven when the bomb went off; we each had a brother who was nineteen. I know how powerful that position is, because I know the way my brother looks up to me. He would do anything I ask. Alan is Air Force Strong, now that he's been through boot camp, so maybe he's different, but a year ago... anything I told him, he would have believed.

I read about Tamerlan recently. I avoided it for a long time, but after a while I wanted to know. What I found was a bully. A boxer who quit but still liked to beat people up. A man who'd scream at the leader of his mosque. Who'd intimidate people in his neighborhood. He had a terrible temper. He assaulted his girlfriend. He was married, but his wife was just another person to bully and abuse. He was a man whose religion—no, not his religion, but his *interpretation* of his religion—wouldn't allow a woman to be his equal.

Maybe that was the biggest difference between him and me, I sometimes think. He had a whipping post. I have a partner.

I go back to those big decisions. Maybe I think about them, because I'm in the process of making them now. I'm at the time in life when you become an adult. When you have to make big decisions to determine who you will be, because not making them becomes a decision in itself.

Tamerlan Tsarnaev... he was too small. He couldn't handle it. He was a loser. He needed to stand up, but he blew everything up instead.

He wasn't mad about our treatment of Muslims. I mean, he was, and I can see why. We've killed kids over there, I can't deny that.

But that was not why Tamerlan set off a bomb at the Boston Marathon. He set off the bomb because his life hadn't worked out yet, and he was afraid to keep trying. He thought the world wasn't fair. He was right: the world isn't fair. Life is tough. There are people committing suicide at factories in China, just so we can have cheap iPhones. That sucks.

But do you blow the whole thing up? No. Hell no. There are other ways. Setting off a bomb, or shooting up an elementary school, doesn't make you bigger. It makes you the smallest kind of person on earth. The kind who has to blame others, because you can't face yourself.

I guess I am angry about that. I'm angry that a loser like Tamerlan Tsarnaev found a way to hurt other people. He's gone, and the only thing he left on this earth was victims.

No, I won't give him that. I'm not his victim. Neither are the Corcorans or the Odoms or all the other people I admire. We're all going to be stronger, even the families of the ones we lost. I won't give in to anger, because being angry will make me more like him. But also because anger means he mattered. And he didn't. His life was nothing.

The victim of his hatred and cowardice, in the end, was his own brother.

I heard the *Rolling Stone* article ended with Dzhokhar crying for two straight days in his hospital room. People were confused by that. They wondered what he was crying about.

I'm not confused. He was a human being. He killed a child. Of course he cried. Why wouldn't he? He was done.

I was at the beach.

And sure, part of my visit to Maine was painful, and part of it was frustrating. I sat at the end of the walk, staring at the beach. I couldn't move in the sand, either in my wheelchair or with my artificial legs. I was stuck, until Uncle Dale scooped me up, put me on his back, and carried me to our blanket, piggyback style.

The day was warm, but the beer was cool. I looked at the water and thought about Mrs. Corcoran, and how she had loved to walk on the beach, and how she cried because she'd never do that again. She was right. Neither of us would ever walk on the beach. That sucked. But with Erin and the Forehead beside me, and a beer in my hand, life was good.

That's what I meant when I said, "He's dead, and I'm still here." I meant that Tamerlan would never feel the sunshine.

I still had people to love.

33.

After the trip to the shore, Erin and I started looking for an apartment in Boston. Living in Boston would make things easier for my physical therapy at Spaulding, and also for Erin to eventually find another job. She didn't want to commute between the city and Chelmsford, and Boston had far more opportunities. Besides, I'd always wanted to move into the city. Erin and I had loved hanging in Brighton before the bombing; we had friends like Michele and Remy there, and favorite coffee shops and restaurants. It seemed ideal. We could rent for a year, and see if it was as perfect as we thought.

It took one apartment-hunting trip to realize it wasn't going to work. Being in the city with Erin was fine, and attending events was always fun, but when I thought about being in an apartment alone, or out on the street trying to get to the store late at night, my heart started to race.

I remembered the words of Commissioner Davis on the morning of the manhunt. "We believe this to be a terrorist. We believe this to be a man *who came here* to kill people."

He was wrong. The Tsarnaev brothers hadn't come here to kill us; they already had been here. Whatever else they were, they were part of us. They were Boston, too.

If it wasn't going to be Boston, we both knew that meant finding a place in Chelmsford. It was a big change for Erin. Her life had been in the city, and even when she moved to Mom's to help me, she always assumed she'd be back. So we took it slow, looking at a few apartments a week. There are nice apartments in Lowell and Chelmsford, mostly in converted mills and factories, but we couldn't find anything we liked.

I don't think our hearts were really in it. Mom's apartment was temporary, even though I had been living there for years. It had always seemed temporary; the place I stayed before my life's big decisions were made. Now it was clear I had outgrown it. I needed to take care of Erin, and myself, by moving on.

I was thinking about the future, something Erin and I had avoided in the months since the bombing. The future—my lifetime of disability—was overwhelming. So we kept our focus on the day ahead. Get better. Get stronger. Do what you need, today, to be normal again.

Whenever people asked what I wanted, that's what I told them, "I just want to be normal."

Again and again, I hear it in interviews and articles: "I just want to be normal." To me, that meant walking. I wanted to be confident enough to walk at the 2014 Boston Marathon: no matter the crowd, no matter the fear or bad memories, I wanted to walk.

I knew that meant meeting each of the shorter goals Michelle set for me. I was using crutches instead of the walker. I had been outside and walked in the grass. I was almost ready for stairs. That was my current goal: to walk up and down a flight of stairs. Beyond that, I tried not to think ahead.

But now that Erin and I were moving into our own space, we had to think about the future. Where were we going to be in five years? What did we want?

What does *normal* really mean?

Erin summarized it best. "There are two ways to go," she said. "We can try to put this behind us. You can go back to Costco, and I can go back to hospital administration, and we can try to live a normal life. Or we can embrace the change, and try to do good."

It was a serious question, and one we still haven't answered. Mom knew what she wanted for me: she wanted me to embrace the opportunity. The idea that her son could be a role model for others, that he could raise money for the needy and inspire those dealing with tragedy—I don't think it was something she ever imagined could happen. When she thought of my future, she had always pictured an engineer with a nice house in North Chelmsford.

But what could I do to help the world?

I had money, but I didn't know what to do with it. I had no idea how to set up a charity. And who would my charity benefit? There were so many people seriously injured who didn't have anyone to help them. I had seen plenty at Spaulding.

There were thousands of children battling cancer. I had met them at charity events.

A chancellor at the University of Massachusetts Lowell had written to me about a scholarship for victims of the bombing. "If in the future, if you look again toward UMass Lowell, please know that we will do everything we can to make this campus a welcoming place for you," the chancellor wrote.

But I didn't need their help now. I had needed it *then*, when I was nobody, and $900 could have changed my life. Should I try to help others in a similar situation?

Erin would have to be involved, of course, in any charity work. I'd be the face; she'd be in charge. But would she be happy? Or did she need her own job, away from Jeff Bauman World?

"You can write a book," Kat suggested.

Ummm...

"It would get your story out, the way you want it told."

But...

"And it could help people. Inspire them."

I'm not so sure...

"And you wouldn't have to talk to the media. Not until the book came out, anyway."

Okay, now you're talking.

Mom loved the idea. Erin wasn't convinced. Actually, that's wrong.

She hated the idea. She's a private person. She didn't want to invite strangers into our lives.

But she could see the advantages, too. She wanted to help people. Erin cares about others more than anyone I've ever known.

And I knew I needed something to do. Maybe I even needed a way to think about what I'd been through. A book wasn't just telling my story. It was putting the story behind me. It was taking all those memories, and putting them in a box, and then shoving that box on the top shelf, where I didn't have to look at it, but where it would always be when I needed it. When I was ready.

As long as it didn't tire me too much, I told Erin, a book might be like therapy.

"It's your decision," Erin said. "I only have one request. If you're going to do it, do it right."

A few days later, Erin and I were having lunch at one of our favorite restaurants, Joe's American Bar and Grill, in downtown Boston. It was her mom's birthday. I knew Erin's mom had taken what happened to me hard, and that she wanted to be a part of my recovery, even if she never asked. So I had invited her to physical therapy with me that morning, then to lunch. The restaurant is on Newbury Street, two blocks from where the bombs went off on Boylston Street. I thought I'd be okay, since those are just regular city blocks now, and they've cleaned up all the blood.

But being in that part of town, I have to admit, made me nervous. It reminded me that evil existed. That terrible things could be done to you when you least expected it. If a bomb could go off on Boylston Street, why not here?

So while I loved the lunch, and especially the company, by the end I was ready to go. But when I asked for the check, the waitress told us it had already been paid.

"By who?" I asked.

"They wanted to remain anonymous."

I gave her the puppy-dog eyes. Who can resist a man in a wheelchair?

"They didn't want to bother you," she said.

"We just want to say thank you."

The waitress laughed. "That's what they wanted me to tell you."

I don't know how to describe it. It was like . . . I was standing in the rain, and a stranger came up and gave me an umbrella, then walked away without a word. Weeks later, I was still thinking about it. About how much small things can mean.

It made me realize that maybe I *could* do the world some good.

34.

Sometime that summer, Kevin mentioned that he would be out of town for a week at the Costco Annual Manager's Conference in Seattle. "I'm gonna be there one year, Heavy Kevy," I joked. "I'm gonna take your job."

Kevin looked at me. "No," he said. "You're going this year, Jeff. I'm going to take you, if you really want to go."

"No, no," I said. "I can't..."

But he was serious, and a few days later, he had tickets for Erin and me. He wanted me to meet the people who had been rooting for me and supporting me. And he wanted them to meet me. He was proud of me, I guess. Not for what I'd been through, but for who I was.

The plane flight proved easier than anticipated. I wore my legs, and except for an excessively intimate fifteen-minute pat-down at airport security, I moved through the airport like anyone else. This was the longest trip I'd been on since I went to Paris and Normandy with my high school friends Pete and Jae when I was twenty-three years old. I had never been this far from Boston with Erin. I was looking forward to getting away. Once we were out of Boston, I could walk down the street without being recognized.

We went for a special dinner the first night with my fellow amputees Byron and Will, along with some of my biggest supporters, like the Costco media buyer, Pennie Clark Ianniciello, who had been sending me care packages since my first week in the hospital. In fact, she was still sending care packages for the people on the fifth floor at Spaulding, even though I was no longer staying there.

Pennie wanted to know everything, so I told her about rehab, Erin, the city of Boston. I told her I was considering writing a book. I was thinking of calling it *Stronger*, because it would be about how the bombing didn't stop me, but made me love my life more.

She encouraged me to do it. "That's the kind of story we want to support," she told me. "An ass-kicker." Pennie was hilarious. We had dinner together three or four times, and I can't even begin to tell you the stories she laid on us, because they'd probably get the book banned from her stores.

After the dinner, we went to Kerry Park for the view, and then the Ferris wheel below Pike Place Market for a sunset ride. Most people went home after the Ferris wheel, but Will and his wife came back to the hotel with us. He brought his guitar, and we jammed for hours.

The next day, I went to corporate headquarters to meet the new CEO, Craig Jelinek, and the former CEO, Jim Sinegal, who was still on the board of directors. Mr. Sinegal had founded and built one of the largest companies in the United States, but his office looked like it belonged to an accountant. Instead of a desk, he had two folding tables, and they were full of papers. The only decoration was an enormous corkboard full of pictures of employees. He had a famous green pen; everyone at Costco talked about getting "green ink," which meant Mr. Sinegal had signed on. For years, he had checked on and approved everything from the mix of candy in the five-pound bags to my top-notch health insurance.

And he was always right.

That night, Mr. Sinegal invited Erin, Byron, and me to sit at the head table with him for the big company dinner. His wife was there, too. They were the nicest people. You would never guess they were worth, like, a hundred million dollars. Mr. Jelinek introduced Byron and me, and he talked about our special bond. Someone later told me Byron hadn't been wearing his legs to work but had started wearing them again after meeting me. We had inspired each other.

The next day, Kevin and his partner took Erin and me on a tour of the city. Kevin had grown up in Washington State, so we met his family, and his sister took us out in her boat so we could view the city from the water. There was a company party at Safeco Field—Huey Lewis and the News! Surprisingly good!—and everyone with legs danced. Everyone at Costco was extraordinary. Everyone. It was an honor to be able to thank them in person, because they had done so much for Erin and me.

But there was one other person I was just as eager to meet.

In July, Erin had showed me her new copy of *Runner's World* magazine. Inside was a picture of a man with no shirt, balanced only on his arms. He was strong. That's the second thing you noticed. The first was that he had no legs. The full-page facing headline said: "Andre Kajlich Is Tougher Than You (He Might Be Happier, Too)."

I read the story immediately. When Andre was twenty-four years old, he was hit by a subway train while attending college in Czechoslovakia. He lost one leg above the knee. He lost his other leg above the hip. These are devastating injuries. Two artificial joints in a leg is hard; three is nearly impossible. But Andre was determined. He not only learned to walk on his hands, he learned to walk on his artificial legs. He got a job at a university and spent his summers working at a camp for teenagers who had lost limbs. He began competing in paratriathlons and was the 2012 Paratriathlete of the Year. The article had been written just after he'd completed the Brazil 135, a 135-mile, three-day ultramarathon, in his wheelchair.

"I want to meet Andre," I told Erin, as soon as Kevin mentioned the trip. Andre was from Edmonds, Washington, but he lived in Seattle. Erin e-mailed *Runner's World*, and to our amazement, Andre e-mailed back. He wanted to meet me, too. So that was what I was thinking as the plane touched down: I'm going to meet Andre Kajlich. Andre is tougher than you.

And happier, too.

We met Andre for dinner one night: Erin, Byron, Pennie, Kevin, and me. He came by himself. That's the first thing I noticed. You could see his artificial legs, but he didn't seem to notice them. To Andre, they were no big deal.

He sat down with a smile. He was very unassuming. He was oozing swag; he just had that air, but he was also humble and down to earth. He asked about everyone, really taking an interest, and when he talked about himself... it wasn't that he believed there was nothing he couldn't do. It was like he never even doubted it. He talked about his work with children, and about the Challenged Athletes Fund, a charity that promoted community among amputees and donated prosthetics to people in need.

"There's a CAF weekend in San Diego next month," he told me. It was a get-together, he explained, for people missing limbs. No pressure, just support. He wanted Byron and me to come.

"Maybe," I said, although I knew another cross-country trip so soon was too much. But I told my newlywed friends, Pat and Jess, about it, and they went. When they came back, they were so excited. They had all these pictures of little kids running around with each other on their artificial legs, having a great time.

Andre was planning to run the Los Angeles and the Boston marathons to raise money for CAF.

"You're going to wheelchair-race two marathons in a month?" Erin asked, impressed.

No, Andre was hoping to complete the Los Angeles Marathon, then wheelchair across the country with a friend to the Boston Marathon, and complete it, too. The races were forty-four days apart. If they made it, it would be the fastest recorded nonmotorized crossing of the United States.

I don't care if he makes it. I really don't. I don't care if he even tries. To dream that big—for it to be in the realm of possibility—is inspiring.

That's what Andre does: he inspires. He's strong in mind and body. Ridiculously good-looking. Highly educated. Smart. Both his parents were doctors. His sister is a famous actress. (And talk about good-looking. Wow, the genes in that family.)

I'm never going to be like Andre. He's a purebred. Top-of-the-line legit.

I'm a mutt.

But that's okay. The mutts are the ones who surprise you.

35.

Back in Boston, I hit the gym hard. I was more tired from the trip to Seattle than I would admit, but I knew there was no time to rest. I was never going to be like Andre, but I had my goals. With Michelle's help, I walked on a sloped surface, and on the grass outside Spaulding. On August 17, four months after losing my legs, I walked for ten straight minutes on a treadmill.

"You're ready to start on stairs," Michelle said.

Now this was progress.

A few days later, I started feeling pain in my right leg. I could tell the fit of my socket wasn't right. A gap had opened at the bottom, between my leg and the plastic, and no matter how much I cinched the Velcro strap, I couldn't get it tight. That caused the rest of the socket to move while I was walking, pinching and rubbing different parts of my thigh.

The fit is important. That's one of the things I remember Byron and Will telling me when I met them back in June. "If you get a good fit on one of your legs, never change it. A good fit is everything."

I talked to Michelle about the problem. She recommended I try an extra sock, which is like putting on an extra pair of underwear if your pants are too big. I mean, really? Erin always carried extra socks in her purse, so I put one on and walked a few steps. It didn't work. The fit was still loose, and now it was pinching at the hip.

"This often happens," Michelle told me. I had sustained massive physical trauma, not just at the point where my legs were ripped off, but throughout my body. My legs were still retaining fluid, and sometimes this fluid moved around.

"Don't worry," Michelle said. "We'll get the prosthetics people down for your next session."

I walked on my crutches between the parallel bars. I stood and made motions like I was swinging an ax over my shoulder, first the right, then the left, focusing on shifting my weight without tipping over. By the time Michelle suggested the stairs, my thighs were barking. I was confident, though, as I walked to the equipment: four wooden stairs that led up to a platform, with four more leading down the other side. It was always in the corner of the gym; I had been watching patients working on it for months.

I didn't make it to the first step. I couldn't raise my foot high enough.

"It's a new motion," Michelle explained. "It's not just lifting. You have to kick your lower leg backward, then pull up your knee, then bring the lower leg forward. That's the only way to clear the riser."

It sounded like what I had been doing for months. Isn't that how you walk? But when I tried to kick my lower leg backward, I couldn't do it.

"Don't worry," Michelle said. "Nobody gets it the first time."

With walking, everything went forward. I shifted my weight slightly, lifted one leg, then swung it in front of me. There was only a slight bend in the knee, and the forward movement contributed to my balance. Everything worked together.

But now I had to lift backward to move forward, throwing everything out of balance.

"Don't be discouraged," Michelle said. "You'll get used to it."

I stared at my foot. I tried to move it backward. Nothing happened. I was prepared for not being able to lift myself up, but I wasn't prepared for that kind of failure. I looked at Erin. I tried one more time, sweat beading on my forehead, but it wasn't to be.

"I can't do it," I said grimly.

Erin put her arm around my waist, while I held on to the railing of the stairs to nowhere.

"There's a reason we wait on stairs," Michelle said.

I didn't talk much on the way home. The realization was sinking in that, for all my progress, I still had a long way to go. *It's only been a few months*, I thought. *Stick with your goals.* But doubt was rattling around in my brain: It's only been a few months, and think about how hard it's been. Now think about the rest of your life.

I went home and sat in my room. I took off my legs. My undercarriage and thighs were sweaty and sore. They were always sweaty and sore. I propped my legs by my bed and started playing *MLB: The Show*. I was playing as a historical All-Star team. I had Pedro on the mound. Nobody could touch Pedro.

I heard Erin rattling around in the kitchen, trying to get dinner together. Mom came in, and I could hear them talking. Rattling around—walking around—and talking. I just wanted to get away. I called a friend, and Erin drove me over and dropped me off so I could watch the Red Sox, have a few beers, and forget.

When she came to pick me up, an hour after midnight, Erin was crying.

"What's the matter?"

She had gone out for a few hours, Erin told me, after dropping me off. She felt good. Relaxed. But as soon as she walked in the door, Mom pounced.

I had found a house I liked online. It was one story, on a hill, with a nice, trimmed front yard. We were scheduled to see it with a real estate agent the next afternoon.

Mom was furious at Erin about the house. She didn't think I could handle a house on a hill. Erin tried to tell her there was no harm in looking.

Mom wouldn't hear it. She accused Erin of pressuring me. She said Erin was getting my hopes up. That the house wasn't realistic.

"He likes it," Erin said. "It's the first house he's actually wanted to see."

"What if he wants to buy it?"

"That's Jeff's decision."

"But he can't handle a house on a hill."

Mom had been home alone, hitting the Cavit. When she was like that, she couldn't stop. She wouldn't let Erin go. "I don't understand why you need a house right now," Mom screamed.

"Jeff's ready to move on."

"He's not ready."

"He's twenty-seven years old."

"He's twenty-seven, but he has no legs."

"So what? He can still do what he wants."

"Why are you pressuring?"

"I'm not pressuring him."

"Why this house?"

"He chose it."

"But it's wrong for him."

"I know that, Patty. I know that. But Jeff has to learn that for himself."

Mom started to protest, but Erin cut her off. "He has to make his own decisions," she said. "I am not going to tell him what to do."

Now, a half hour later, Erin was in the car outside my friend's house, shaking. This didn't happen in her family, she said. I knew it was probably the worst fight of her life.

"I can't do it, Jeff," she said. "I can't take this." She paused. "I'm not even sure she's going to remember what happened."

"Drive me home," I said.

It was almost two in the morning, but Mom was still up, like I knew she'd be. I laid into her. I yelled at her like I never had before. She yelled back, at first, but eventually she backed down. She just... gave in.

I went to bed an hour later, but I couldn't sleep. I lay in bed beside Erin, staring at the ceiling. I hadn't slept for months, but somehow, this was different. This hurt more.

The next day, Erin and I went to see the house. It wasn't right for me.

36.

In mid-August, Big D drove me to Watertown. Erin had lived only a few blocks away, across the Charles River in Brighton, and we'd often come over to Watertown for shopping or dinner. I liked it in Watertown, a working-class suburb that had been spruced up in the last decade. It was odd to think that here, surrounded by close-packed houses and new shopping centers, the bombers had made their stand.

I had stayed in touch with the Watertown police since meeting them at the Bruins game. We texted every few days, and I had run into their chief of police, Ed Deveau, at a charity event and then a Harry Connick Jr. concert earlier in the summer. The Charles River Country Club in nearby Newton had offered the department free golf and swimming for the day, in appreciation of their heroism, and Chief Deveau insisted I come. I was part of it, he told me. We wouldn't have caught them without you.

My swing was a little rusty, so I passed on the golf. Big D and I met them later on the patio of the clubhouse. The first person I saw was Vincent D'Onofrio. I'm never star-struck—okay, with Pedro, only Pedro—but...Vincent D'Onofrio! I'd watched him on *Law & Order: Criminal Intent* a hundred thousand times.

Turned out he was friends with Chief Deveau. I assumed it was a police research kind of friendship, but who knows? Chief Deveau was a lifer. He had been in the trenches for years, but he had the air of a politician, in a good way. He had class.

The chief invited me right over to his table, and after a bit of conversation, he introduced some of his men. There was a lot of misinformation about the shootout circulating. Even I had questions when the story broke: How did Dzhokhar escape a whole police force? How did he manage to hit his own brother with their car, the official cause of Tamerlan's death?

I've pieced it together, mostly by listening to the stories of the Watertown cops and the help of a few articles and news programs. This isn't how they told it to me. This is my smoothed-out version of all the bits and pieces I put together that afternoon and over time. Those guys tell stories about that day—I think they feel compelled to tell stories, to try to sort it out—but they don't brag. Not at all. They are proud, but they are humble, too. I think they still find it hard to believe what happened: that a typical sighting of a stolen car had turned into four hundred bullets fired and three bombs detonated in five minutes on a quiet residential street.

Officer Joe Reynolds had spotted the stolen car coming down Dexter Avenue from the direction of Cambridge. He thought it was an ordinary carjacking. "They always have those in Cambridge," Chief Deveau joked.

This was three days after the bombing, and maybe six hours after the first surveillance photos of the suspects were released. MIT police officer Sean Collier had been gunned down in Cambridge two hours before. Boston was on high alert; thousands of tips had been called in to hotlines. But Boston is a city, and there is always crime, even that week. A 7-Eleven was robbed near the time and place of the carjacking, for instance, but it was totally unrelated. There was nothing to indicate this was anything other than kids out for a joy ride.

The driver obviously saw the patrol car coming toward him, though, because he suddenly turned onto Laurel, a small side street, and turned off his engine. Officer Reynolds drove past the intersection, called in the stolen vehicle, then swung around and slowly rolled into position on Laurel Street, a few houses behind the stolen car, to wait for backup.

Then Tamerlan stepped out of a second car and started shooting. He was walking toward the police cruiser, only two car lengths away, and calmly firing into the windshield. Officer Reynolds ducked, put his cruiser in reverse, and hit the gas pedal hard. A round went through the windshield, shattering the glass in his face.

His backup, Sergeant John MacLellan, felt something sizzle past his ear as soon as he turned onto Laurel. He was still trying to figure out what was happening when a second bullet hit the headrest an inch from his other ear. He threw open the door to give himself room and ducked behind it for cover.

The two patrol cars, going in opposite directions, had wound up side by side. The officers were pinned down, only a few feet apart, with only their pistols. Tamerlan was closing, and the brothers were firing so many rounds into the cruisers that they couldn't even lift their heads to assess the situation. So Sergeant MacLellan reached in, put his cruiser in drive, and let it roll down the street toward Tamerlan. Both brothers turned to fire at it. Then Tamerlan ran for cover, and his brother threw a pipe bomb, blowing out the car windows. By the time the cruiser bumped lightly into a car parked in a driveway five houses down, Officer Reynolds and Sergeant MacLellan had taken cover behind a tree.

I have never visited the bomb site on Boylston Street, where my legs were turned to applesauce. I've planned to three times, but I've always found an excuse to back out. One day I'll go there, before next year's marathon, for sure, just not quite yet.

But I visited the site of the shootout. I've seen that tree. It's six inches around at most and pocked with bullet holes. The officers must have crapped their pants when they returned the next day and saw how small it was.

"I thought it was a sequoia," Sergeant MacLellan said. "I thought it was big as a house."

Four guns were blazing when Sergeant Jeff Pugliese arrived on the scene. He had been leaving the police station in his family minivan when he heard the call. He saw the Tsarnaevs hidden behind their cars, with the two officers pinned down, so he raced around the back of the nearest house to get behind them. He had to climb two fences in the process. Sergeant Pugliese is a thirty-three-year veteran, so he's no youngster, "but I vaulted those fences," he said.

The Tsarnaevs were firing rounds at a ferocious clip. They threw two more pipe bombs. The first blew out car windows and shook Sergeant MacLellan so hard that his eyeballs bounced around in their sockets. The second was a dud. As Tamerlan covered him, Dzhokhar ran out and placed a pressure-cooker bomb, like the one that destroyed my legs, in the middle of the street. That was when the people in the surrounding houses stopped taking pictures, because everybody scattered when they saw that fat bomb. Officer Reynolds managed to get behind the nearest house, but Sergeant MacLellan, still trying to recover from the concussion of the pipe bomb, was trapped in the kill zone behind the tree.

Something happened. Probably the top slid off the pressure cooker before detonation, but nobody is sure. The bomb exploded, but instead of blasting out, the shrapnel blew straight up. As it rained down, Sergeant Pugliese took up position twenty feet from the brothers and started skip-firing bullets—he was actually bouncing them off the ground so they would go under their car.

Tamerlan was hit in the leg. He went down. For a moment, it was quiet. Then, without warning, Tamerlan charged from behind the car straight at Sergeant Pugliese, firing as he came. It was like that scene in *Pulp Fiction*, when the kid charges Vincent and Jules in the apartment. Tamerlan was ten feet away; he put bullet holes in the wall right where Sergeant Pugliese was crouching, but the sergeant wasn't hit.

"Freeze," Sergeant MacLellan yelled, charging at Tamerlan with his gun drawn. He was out of bullets, but Tamerlan didn't know that, so Sergeant MacLellan jerked his arm like he was firing. Tamerlan turned, then realized he too was out of bullets, right before Sergeant Pugliese hit him full force from behind and knocked him to the ground. Both officers jumped on top of him. Tamerlan had been shot multiple times by Sergeant Pugliese, but real police bullets don't have the stopping power of movie bullets. Tamerlan was badly wounded, but he fought like an animal.

Meanwhile, two other police cruisers had arrived, blocking the intersection of Dexter and Laurel. By then, Dzhokhar had jumped in the stolen car. The other end of Laurel was open, but instead of escaping, he flipped a U-turn and floored it back toward the two officers struggling with Tamerlan. His intention, apparently, was to run them down, but at the last minute the officers rolled out of the way, and he slammed into his brother instead. The car dragged the body half a block, before plowing into a police cruiser and escaping into Watertown.

And still, when they came with the cuffs, Tamerlan struggled. Despite his fatal wounds, it took three officers to hold him. It was only after he was finally cuffed that they realized Dicky Donohue, a Massachusetts Bay Transportation Authority officer who had just arrived on the scene, was down.

"You'll find a hundred guys that say they were there," one of the cops on the patio said. "But we know the truth. There were only eight. And except for Dicky and his partner, they were all Watertown."

"Three Watertown cops took the older bastard down," someone else piped in. "But it took twenty-five hundred to arrest his little brother." As it turned out, Dzhokhar was only ten blocks away, hiding in a boat.

I remember shaking Sergeant MacLellan's hand that day. He was one of the officers I had met at the Bruins game, and we had been texting for weeks, but I had no idea until that golf outing what he had done. Can you imagine a more unlikely handshake? The guy who was standing closest to a bomb, and the guy who hid behind a sapling in a gun fight.

Sergeant Pugliese was also there, looking nothing like a guy who could vault a fence. Only when the adrenaline was pumping, I guess.

Dicky Donohue was there with his wife and two young children.

He had been in critical condition for a long time, and he was still walking with a cane. He didn't remember anything about that night, but he knew who had saved him.

"These guys are heroes," he said.

"We were doing our jobs," John MacLellan said.

"It's amazing more people weren't hurt," the chief said. Everyone nodded in agreement. Hundreds of bullets had been fired, bombs had been thrown, and only Tamerlan had died.

We were all quiet for a second, thinking about that. Despite what the movies suggest, shootouts like that never happen. "We had almost seventy-two years of experience on that street," the chief said, "and nobody had fired their gun in the line of duty. Not even once."

"It's over now," someone said, raising a beer. "To Jeff."

"To Sean Collier."

"To Dicky."

"To the Watertown PD," I said. "Thank you."

37.

That same weekend, I went to my nephew Cole's birthday party in Aunt Jenn's backyard. It was the middle of August, and it was hot. The Dog Days, they call them in the baseball season, a hundred degrees, one hundred twenty games down, and forty-two to go. The Yankees had collapsed, and the Sox were battling for the best record in the league. Koji Uehara was killing it in the bullpen, and Big Papi was ripping, but I couldn't get excited about a possible World Series. Playoffs, sure, but no team goes from worst to first in a year, not even a team like this one built on grit, togetherness, and bat-shit crazy. They ground out small victories, day after day. They grew beards in some sick show of solidarity. And I don't mean nice, trimmed beards. I mean face muffins.

I don't like the Sox, a friend from New York texted me. But those Amish guys are pretty good.

Hard to believe that only a year ago, I'd introduced Erin to my family after Cole's party. Now she was practically a member of the family, and no one could imagine a celebration without Carlos and Kevin. I watched them chatting with each other, two of the many people who had come through for me. I watched Cole, Big D, and Sully jumping in the bounce house. It seemed impossible: not just jumping, which was of course impossible for me, but being on the sidelines like that, doing my own thing and having fun, without anybody watching.

A few days before the party, Cole had set up a lemonade stand for me. "I'm going to give Uncle Jeff all the money," he told Aunt Jenn. Aunt Jenn lived on a main road between the highway and downtown North Chelmsford. It was two lanes, but there was a lot of traffic. Cole put up the banner that had been across the highway on the day I left Spaulding:

Welcome Home, Jeff. Bauman Strong.

I was sick of that banner, but Cole was so happy to be helping his uncle, just like everyone else. He raised $120 selling lemonade. A few of the neighbors gave him $20 and told him to keep the change.

He gave me the money at the party: $60. He had decided, since he did all the work, and it was his ninth birthday and all, that splitting the money was fair.

"Thank you, Forehead," I said.

I could tell how much stronger I was because it was so easy to wrestle him, even from my wheelchair. Cole is so hyperactive, he can get past most defenses. But now when I held him at arm's length, he couldn't get close.

"Go get yourself a Snickers, Forehead," Uncle Bob joked. "We're talking here." Did I mention that Cole has a peanut allergy? Uncle Bob was shameless.

Cole wandered off, although not for a Snickers. Uncle Bob and I stuck to our hot dogs and beer. Around my family, it was mostly like the old days. They were used to me, and they treated me like they always had. But even at Cole's party, there were people who hadn't met me before. Who cried when they saw me and wanted to shake my hand.

I thought about the Watertown party. One of the detectives had come up to me later in the evening. "I texted my wife you were here," he said, wiping tears from his eyes. "She wanted me to tell you she loves you. That she thinks about you every day."

Are you kidding me? Look over there, that's Sergeant John MacLellan. That guy refused to move from behind a tree so he could get a better shot at the bombers. He charged a guy with a gun without knowing the guy was out of bullets. After the shootout, they found bits of shrapnel in his bulletproof vest.

John MacLellan is a hero. John MacLellan deserves to be on a postage stamp.

Me? I can't even climb a set of stairs.

I looked at Aunt Jenn's aboveground pool, with its five steps. I had been working for four months, killing myself with leg lifts and walking practice. I had been working on stairs for two solid weeks, and still those steps were insurmountable. I couldn't have gone into the pool unless I'd been willing to use my arms to crawl, and I wasn't in the mood to sit on the ground and haul myself up like a gimp.

Besides, I'd gone to Mrs. Corcoran's sister's house the week before. It was the first time we'd seen each other since Spaulding. Mrs. Corcoran was adjusting to her new legs. Sydney had gone to her senior prom, where she was voted Prom Queen. It was a beautiful day. Erin and I were in her sister's pool, having a great time, laughing and wrestling, when suddenly I went under. Somehow, I got pushed toward the bottom. I couldn't get up. My arms were pinned, and I had no way to kick to the surface.

In a second, I went from happy to helpless. From hope to just... pathetic.

Even worse, the dunk screwed up my hearing. My ears had been improving all summer, but the water pressure screwed up something inside. A week later, in Aunt Jenn's backyard, the party sounded like a wall of sound.

I took a sip of my beer.

I eyed the stairs to the aboveground pool.

I thought about the back kick, the first step in climbing stairs. Michelle had introduced a new piece of equipment: a piece of paper. She slid it under the foot I was trying to kick back. It was supposed to eliminate friction. I focused on putting my weight on the paper, then kicking it backward. If I could make the paper fly, Michelle said, I would have the correct motion.

How hard was it to make a piece of typing paper fly?

Two weeks, and the paper never flew.

38.

Jules from United Prosthetics met me at Spaulding. She had checked my legs many times before, so I knew her well. "How was your wedding?" I asked.

"Oh, you know," she said. "Perfect."

She went to help another patient. By the time she came back, I was in the middle of my session with Michelle. I had walked back and forth using the parallel bars four times, turning around at the end each time.

"I'm tired," I told Jules. "More tired than I used to be."

"It's the loose fit," she said. "Even a little slippage makes it harder to do the same work. You're probably using four or five times more effort than before. Do you have any pain?"

"Lots."

"Where?"

"Everywhere," I said. "It moves around."

"Have you tried an extra sock?"

Michelle had already suggested the extra sock. "It pinches my hip."

"We can cut it down," Jules said. She explained again that my leg was changing shape. Some areas were bigger than when the socket was created. Others were smaller. Because of the trauma, and the long process of healing, my thighs would probably keep changing shape for the next year. "We can cut the sock to fill in the smaller parts. We can also stuff pieces down in the bottom of the socket, to fill in the gaps at the end of your leg. That's where you're really losing energy."

Erin handed Jules a couple extra socks, and she cut them into shape. I was pissed. These were $100,000 legs, and the best way to correct the fit was to cut some socks and jam cloth into the end of them?

"Can't I get a new socket?"

"It will take a few weeks," Jules said, handing me the second sock to roll onto my left leg. "And your leg is changing shape fast. If we can make this work, it's a better option."

I fit the socket on my leg, then tightened it with the Velcro strap.

"What about the suction cup?"

I hated the Velcro straps. I had a one-hundred-adjustments-per-second microchip in my artificial knee, and I secured it to my leg with the stuff little kids used to hold on their shoes. I wanted to move up to the suction version, which adhered through compression between my leg and the bottom of my socket. Even that seemed like something a middle school kid would come up with for a science fair, but everyone said it was far more effective.

"That's not a good idea," Michelle said.

"We prefer to wait for your leg to settle into shape," Jules confirmed, feeling my socket like a shoe salesman might feel the foot inside a new shoe. "If the fit isn't perfect, the suction won't work. Take a few steps."

I stood up and walked. The leg felt like deadweight. It was lift, clunk. Lift, clunk. All the technology, and all I really had was a door with a hinge attached to my leg.

"Does it hurt now?" she asked.

"It hurts a lot."

Jules stared at the leg. "Let me think about it," she said finally. "I'm going to ask for second opinions at the office. We'll get you sorted."

I stood still while she adjusted my legs with electronic readings and small screwdrivers. Jules had a whole case full of tiny tools.

"He's having trouble with the back kick," Michelle told her.

"Have you tried a piece of paper?"

Geez, I thought, could this get any more high-tech? Freaking typing paper.

Jules made more adjustments, loosening (or possibly tightening) something to make the kick easier. Each person was different. It took hundreds of adjustments, over several months, to find the right balance.

After the adjustments, I walked to the stairs and pulled myself to the top. Michelle stood behind and held me, so I wouldn't tip backward. I couldn't kick and bend my knee enough to keep my weight forward.

At the top, I turned to face down the stairs. Michelle showed me how to place my foot halfway over the edge, then lean forward and bend my other leg, then drop it down. It was scary. I couldn't feel the stair, because artificial legs are basically stilts, and I could see the drop. It felt like I was falling. Instead, the leg kept locking. I couldn't get my foot down to the next step.

"That's the safety mechanism," Jules said.

We tried again and again, working on adjustments. Jules tightened and loosened. I tried to keep my weight and positioning just right. But if the angle of my standing foot changed too much or too quickly, the leg locked. Or if my weight went too far forward . . . or if I didn't bend the standing leg correctly . . . or my feet were on different planes. I don't know. There were a hundred different problems to solve.

Just give me the pirate leg, I thought. Just give me the wooden peg, like those old-timers on the wall back at the office.

Two weeks before, Erin and I had finally found a house. It was a one-story ranch on a flat lot. The floors were wooden, easier for me than carpet, and the doorways were wide enough for a wheelchair. Uncle Bob lived a few blocks away, and it was ten minutes to Mom's. It was ideal, except for three small steps outside the front door.

"I'm going to walk up those steps," I told Erin, when our offer was accepted. "You won't even need to help me. I'm going to walk up those steps and into our new life on my own."

The marathon was eight months away, and walking without crutches, especially in front of thousands of people, still seemed like a step too far. I needed a more manageable goal. Something to focus my mind.

The stairs at the house were perfect. Two weeks ago, I hadn't even wondered if it would happen. I had known I would walk up those stairs.

Now I wasn't so sure. I hadn't made progress in weeks. I had stopped wearing my legs, except to Spaulding. If the next month went like the last one, Erin would have to carry me up those stairs. And looking failure in the face like that, setting a goal I might not achieve...it was something I'd been trying to avoid for a long time.

"You'll get it, Jeff, don't worry," Michelle said, putting her arm around my sweaty back and helping me down. "It just takes practice, like riding a bike. Once you've mastered it, you'll be able to do it in your sleep."

I didn't say anything. I just grabbed my crutches and walked toward the door with Erin. It was time to go home.

39.

We went to Manchester, New Hampshire, to meet my dad, Big Csilla, my brother Chris, and my stepsister Erika. Dad had been pressuring me to come to Concord and see him, but his house wasn't wheelchair accessible, and even though Erin did the driving (another issue), sitting that long in one position bothered my legs.

"Just a quick trip, son," he said, every time we talked on the phone. "You used to come up all the time."

People from his church were donating their time and supplies to make his house better for me: a wheelchair ramp and porch, the new first-floor bedroom. He wanted those people to meet me. "It's so easy," my dad kept saying. "Why aren't you coming to see me?" He didn't understand that things that used to be easy, and that I used to do all the time, were the worst for me now. They reminded me how different my life had become.

So we met halfway, in Manchester, New Hampshire, at a comedy club. Erika knew the comedian performing that night. He was funny. We laughed and had a good time. Afterward, he came over and bought us drinks. I'd been pretty tight with my drinking since my injuries. I always had a few at charity events, to help with my social anxiety. But I didn't drink casually anymore, and I never drank more than a beer or three (or maybe four). When I was drunk, emotions came up that I couldn't control.

At the club, though, things got a little tipped. The manager kept offering us free shots of tequila, a form of kindness that had become common since my injuries, but this time I kept drinking them. I can't tell you why. I don't know if it was because I was having a good time

(I was), or because I was frustrated and in pain (I was that, too), or both. After a while, it didn't matter. If you have enough drinks, you have the next one just because it's there. By the time Erin and I left, I was drunk.

Erin usually didn't drink, but she'd put down a few shots. She didn't feel comfortable driving back to Chelmsford, so she suggested sobering up at Lindsay's house. Lindsay was a friend of hers who lived in Manchester.

"I want to go home," I said.

"It will be fun, Jeff," she said. "You know how much Lindsay loves you."

I knew how tough Erin's social life had been since her move to Chelmsford. She hadn't even seen Remy and Michele in a month. Remy had no permanent damage from the bombing. Michele would have permanent scars on her legs and, because of her Achilles tendon damage, she would never be able to jump off her left leg. Michele didn't seem too concerned about that.

"No," I said, "I want to go home."

"I don't feel comfortable driving, Jeff."

"Just take me home."

"I'm sorry. I shouldn't have drank so much."

"Call me a cab," I said. "I'll take a cab to Chelmsford."

"Jeff…"

"Call me a helicopter."

"Jeff…"

"I want a damn helicopter ride home. I can afford it. You know that, right? I can afford a goddamn helicopter ride."

By then, Erin had pulled up in front of Lindsay's house. When I saw it, I lost my shit. It was a hundred-year-old, two-story Victorian, the kind you see all over New England. You had to climb five or six steps just to get to the front door, and I could tell from the street, even in the dark, that those stairs were warped and full of splinters.

"No."

"Please, Jeff."

"No. I am not doing this."

"This is my friend—"

"No," I screamed.

"I need—"

"No," I screamed again, punching my fist into the dashboard. I hit the radio, and the faceplate shattered. I could see the lights in the console flash and go out, but I couldn't feel any pain.

Erin got out of the car and went inside. I knew she was crying. I almost didn't care. I just wanted to be home. But I was stuck in a car I couldn't drive, in the dark, in New Hampshire. Somehow, I managed to haul myself up the stairs and into the house. I remember drinking more. Lindsay made me a cup of coffee, and I remember angrily punching it out of her hand. At one point, I tried to climb the stairs to the second floor. Erin was up there. Each stair had a hard lip that stuck out, battering me as I hauled myself up with my arms. There was a turn in the middle. I didn't make it to the top. I remember lying on the steps, exhausted and ashamed. I knew this would happen. I knew, as soon as I saw the house, that I'd be crawling on the floor.

I hated, right then, but I'm not sure exactly what.

In the end, we slept over. But I couldn't sleep. I had bad nightmares about applesauce and missing legs and the pool of blood. I heard the explosion. I smelled it, like I always did at my worst moments. I tossed on the floor. I lay awake, watching the ceiling spin. At 4:00 in the morning, I pulled myself to the refrigerator for a bottle of water. It was one of those fridges with the freezer on the bottom. Even sitting up, I couldn't reach the shelves.

I grabbed the refrigerator handle and pulled myself onto my legs. I was standing now, without my prosthetics. My weight was driving down on the ends of my femurs. It was like jamming your elbows into the ground and lifting your body with them. I wanted to scream, and maybe I should have. Maybe that was what I needed.

Everything hurt that night. Everything. But the water saved me, because the next morning, it was just my legs that were killing me, and not my head.

———————

We woke up late. It was so late, in fact, that our breakfast was lunch at Taco Bell. "You need to find a way to deal with your emotions," Erin said, as she watched me crunch into a taco wrapped in a Dorito.

"I know."

"You can't let everything build up."

"I know," I said. "I'm sorry."

It was a long ride back to Chelmsford, especially since the radio wasn't working. It had broken when I punched it, something I only hazily remembered. There were a lot of details I didn't remember from the night before: things I'd said to Erin, things I'd said about the bombing and my legs.

"You need to talk to me," Erin said. "And not just when you've been drinking. You need to talk with me when you're sober, too."

But I didn't. I couldn't.

Back at the apartment, Erin packed her things. Before we left for the comedy show she had already planned to stay at her parents' house for a few days. Our house closing was supposed to be the following week, but it had been pushed back for the third time. When Erin heard the news, she said she needed to go home. For a haircut. Her friend was getting married the next weekend, and she was in the wedding. She had to get her dress fitted, organize our overnight trip, coordinate reception details, and help me with my outfit. Because of the bulkiness of my sockets, none of my long pants would fit over my thighs.

"I'm wearing my penguin shorts," I finally told her. "Who is going to complain?"

I knew things were unresolved when she left, and I knew that was because of me. I sat in Mom's apartment for most of the next two days, mostly alone, playing *Battlefield 4* and thinking on and off about Manchester. Erin wanted me to be more open with my emotions, but I'd never been that way. Before Erin, I hadn't even known it was possible to trust someone that much.

I'd always kept my emotions to myself.

"I'm the only one he ever gets mad at," I heard Erin tell someone once.

It was true. And Erin was the only person I was ever sad around, too.

With everyone else, I tried to be the positive one, the person who picked up the mood, who assured the world that everything was fine. With Erin, I realized, it had always been the other way around. On top of everything else, I had relied on her to do that for me.

It was a heavy burden; I knew this from experience. Especially after five months of carrying it. Especially now that my legs weren't fitting right, and I couldn't walk stairs, and I was beginning to wonder if I'd ever live another day without pain.

Could Erin really be happy with a husband like me? Could we ever really have a normal life together?

I didn't want to think those thoughts. I didn't know how to handle them. So I sat on my bed with my PlayStation, shooting enemy soldiers in the back of the head and trying to let the frustrations—with my legs, with the situation—fall apart around me.

Eventually, I had to get up. I had a fund-raiser that night for the Never Quit Foundation, a charity that benefited children with cancer. I dragged myself out of bed and into the shower. I made myself look handsome and happy.

Let's hit it, I texted Big D and Sully, when my boys were finally off work.

An hour later, we rolled up to the House of Blues, where the charity event was being held. The publicist, who had talked with Erin about a hundred times, was waiting for us out front.

"Park right there," she said, indicating a no-parking zone right next to the door. "You have a handicapped sticker, right?"

"I'm not handicapped," I said.

"Oh my God, Jeff, I am so sorry. That was so stupid. I just..."

"I'm kidding," I said, as Big D cracked up. "I am totally handicapped. But I haven't gotten around to getting a sticker."

It was a *Hollywood Square*–style event, featuring a tic-tac-toe board with nine local celebrities in the squares. It was sponsored by Red Sox pitcher Jon Lester, who was diagnosed with cancer during his rookie season in 2006. He and his wife were the contestants. Several Red Sox players were in the squares: John Lackey, Ryan Dempster, Salty. The event was held on a Monday, since that was the team's only day off for weeks. They had played an away game the night before, and the team plane had arrived back in town at 4:00 that morning.

"I only got three hours' sleep," Salty told me, as we chilled at the bar. I didn't tell him that for me, three hours was a good night.

The bar was free, so Big D brought me drinks, while I sat in my wheelchair in a crowd, shaking hands. Carlos and I were the "celebrities" in the bottom right square (the other rows weren't wheelchair accessible), and I needed lubrication to make jokes in front of a crowd of a few hundred people. By the time we took our seats, I was nicely toasted.

"Why does everyone have a last name except Jeff and Carlos?" Dempster said as he looked over the game board. "It just says 'Jeff and Carlos.'"

"Yeah," I joked. "If they can fit 'Saltalamacchia' on Salty's sign, they can fit anything."

"In this town," someone replied, "Jeff and Carlos don't need last names."

Three rounds of Hollywood Squares later, we hit the after party. It must have been sponsored by Smirnoff or something, because the vodka was flowing. I was laughing and having a good time when Big D grabbed me by the shoulder.

"Don't eat the nachos," he said, before rushing off to the snack table. I looked over and saw Sully, smashed on free vodka, trying to shovel a handful of chili-cheese chips into his face. Topping was falling off the chips back into the pile, and the whole wad collapsed out of his hand just before Derek could drag him away.

"Don't eat the nachos," I yelled to Salty. He was standing next to me, but the music was loud.

"Why?" he yelled.

I shook my head. "You don't want to know."

"Centerfolds," I yelled to Big D a few minutes later. He was in the corner with his arms crossed, watching me. It sucks to be the sober driver.

Salty and the other Sox begged off, because of their late flight and lack of sleep, so Sully, Big D, and I ended up on our own at Boston's most famous strip club at 1:30 on a Monday night. I told Erin this might happen, since I'd had free Centerfolds passes for weeks. She'd given her blessing to a boys' night out.

I still can't believe they let us in. I couldn't stop talking smack. "Nacho Man Sully Savage," I kept yelling at Sully, who was passed out in the backseat. "Wake up, Nacho Man!"

It looked like Sully was down for good, but his adrenaline kicked in when he saw the pole. I wrangled a handful of ones, passed them around to my friends, and zoned out. It was only my second time in a strip club in my life, but I liked it, maybe too much.

The fact is, I had seen something in Erin's face on the drive back to Chelmsford, something I was trying to ignore. It wasn't that she was exhausted and overwhelmed. I already knew that. It was that she was afraid.

She wasn't afraid of me. She was afraid *for* me.

No, she was afraid for us.

When we woke up on the morning of the Boston Marathon, Erin and I had known what our lives would be like. Not the details, but the general outline.

Now...we didn't know anything. How long would my recovery take? How healthy would I ever be? How were we going to manage the kids, the cars, the jobs, the emotions? How would we deal with the daily grind of the rest of our lives?

Of course Erin was afraid. So was I.

And I didn't want to think about that. I wanted to play *Battlefield 4*. I wanted to listen to a functioning radio. I wanted to spend two hours handing dollar bills to nearly naked women. Strippers don't make you feel uncomfortable about your legs.

"Nacho Man Sully Savage," I yelled across the room. "You need some bills, Nacho Man?"

Sully smiled, gave me a thumbs-up, and nearly passed out.

40.

When I was twelve, Aunt Karen, Big D's mom, was diagnosed with esophageal cancer. It was devastating, especially because it happened so fast. We were out for dinner one night, and Aunt Karen had trouble swallowing. When it didn't get better, she went to her doctor. The next day, she was admitted to Brigham and Women's Hospital. Two weeks before, she seemed fine. Now she was going to die.

Her illness was one of the reasons Mom and I lived with Uncle Bob for a while, and why Big D and I spent a few months living in Aunt Jenn's condo. My family had always taken care of each other. Not just Mom when the money was tight, but also her special-needs sister, Caroline, who lived with Aunt Jenn and who gave me the best back rubs while I was in the hospital. As soon as we heard the cancer diagnosis, everyone changed their lives around so we could take care of Aunt Karen and her family.

She survived, but she lost her vocal cords. For ten years, Aunt Karen has barely been able to make a sound. At first, that scared me. How could something so horrible happen so fast? How was I supposed to respond when I couldn't understand what Aunt Karen was trying to tell me? I loved being with Aunt Karen, but it made me uncomfortable, too. She was different now—she was different from the rest of us, but also from herself—and every time I talked with her, I was reminded of that.

Those days are long gone now. These days, it's easy to communicate with Aunt Karen. We're used to her limitations, so we don't notice them, and she's developed a way to communicate with whispers, hand gestures, and facial expressions.

These days, Aunt Karen is an inspiration. She texts me all the time.

I'm proud of you, she writes. I'm proud of the way you are handling this.

We don't talk or text about what it's like to be different. I know it bothered her at first, to be out in public without her voice. She was self-conscious. Waitresses would ask for her order, and she'd struggle to respond. A stranger would ask for directions, and she could only point and shake her head. People stared at her as she struggled, like she was some sort of freak.

But if they do that anymore, Aunt Karen doesn't notice. She's comfortable with who she is. Someone asked me how it was around her now, and I shrugged. "I don't think about it," I said. "It's normal to me."

That's what inspires me. When I see Aunt Karen, I realize that one year—if that's how long it takes me to walk—isn't that long. Right now, I don't feel comfortable with myself. I feel self-conscious. My legs hurt. But that doesn't mean I won't feel comfortable in the future. If it takes a few years to accept myself, then so be it. That's no big deal. I just have to keep working. I may be frustrated this week, but I'll be fine next month. Or tomorrow.

I'll always be different. That's my life. But that doesn't mean I'm not normal.

Sometimes, in this process, this public life, I feel like I'm being used. Did the Boston Bruins really want to do something nice for Jeff Bauman the human being? Or did they want him to be a prop? Something they could use to make a crowd of people cheer?

Boston Medical called me around the time of the Nacho Man incident. Or more accurately, they called Erin, again and again, before finally getting to me. Kenny Chesney had given a large donation to the hospital for their work with bombing victims, and he was going to be in town for a charity benefit concert. They asked me and several other bombing survivors to meet with him.

I have nothing against Kenny Chesney. I'm sure he's a nice guy. In fact, I know he's a nice guy, because his charity, Spread the Love, has helped me and a lot of other survivors, too. But I didn't want to meet with him or attend the concert. I wasn't in the right place at that time, in my mental or physical life.

The publicist at BMC insisted. The hospital was going to film the meeting; she wanted me there. It was implied, almost, that I owed the hospital this for saving my life. It's true, they saved my life. I love Boston Medical Center. But they are a hospital. Isn't that what they do?

But more than that, it was like I wasn't even a person. Not a real person, anyway, one who struggled and became frustrated and sometimes wanted to withdraw for a while. I was just a gift they were giving Kenny Chesney, to prove his donation had been well spent.

Look at Jeff, isn't he adorable? Look at Jeff, isn't he brave? Look at Jeff, he's a symbol. He's a marketing tool.

I don't mind that. I really don't. Especially for a good cause like BMC. And especially for my city. I try to do as much as I can, as often as I can. But when it's not my choice...when it feels like I have to, because I owe them, and if I'm hurting and unable, then I'm ungrateful...

Sometimes, when that happens, I just want to quit. I want to disappear.

But then someone will come up to me on the street and ask, "I don't mean to intrude but...can I hug you?"

Or Aunt Karen will text me: I'm proud of you.

Or I'll go to something truly special, like the ceremony on September 11 at the Massachusetts State House. Carlos was being honored with the Madeline Amy Sweeney Award for Civilian Bravery, and he asked me to attend. The award was named for a flight attendant on the airplane that had taken off from Boston and was crashed by terrorists into the World Trade Center. Her daughter, who was six at the time, was at the ceremony. One of the national guardsmen Carlos had been at the marathon to support helped present the award.

"I accept this on behalf of everyone who has had a child die," Carlos said, when they gave him the award.

He was thinking of his own sons. But he was talking about me, too. Carlos has never thought of me as an opportunity. He has never asked anything from me. To him, I was always somebody's son.

That's why I'll do anything for him. Not just because we're friends, but because he treats me like a human being. I don't feel like a prop with Carlos, and I don't feel like a guy who lost his legs. Do you know what I feel like?

I feel like myself.

41.

 Let's go to the Java Room for breakfast," I said to Erin. It was Wednesday morning, two days after my adventure at Centerfolds. She had returned late the previous evening, and of course I had been up. I'd been up all night, but this time, I'd spent most of it thinking.

"Are you sure?" Erin said. I rarely suggested going anywhere, especially for breakfast. I wasn't a morning person.

"I feel like stretching my legs."

"Jeff…"

I was supposed to wear my legs for at least an hour every day. But because of the pain, I hadn't worn them in a week. Just seeing them leaning in the corner had depressed me.

"Yep," I said. "Let's strap 'em on."

Mom had bought me some new shoes at the outlet mall: New Balances (not a pun) to replace my dark blue Nikes. They were wider, she said, so they would be better for my balance.

I lifted one of my legs and looked at them. "I don't like these shoes," I said. "They're ugly. I'm switching back to my Nikes."

So I did. I put the Nikes on my artificial feet, and the extra socks on my legs. Then we rode over to the Java Room in Uncle Bob's Jetta. Both Erin and I had old cars in lousy shape, so she'd been driving Uncle Bob's car since she'd moved to Chelmsford. His radio still played, but we couldn't change the channel or turn down the volume. I knew I had to get it fixed. I went to the dealership for the repair, and I actually ended up buying Erin a used Volkswagen Tiguan, too. (Got a great deal.) So Uncle Bob got his car back in one piece, and Erin and I got our first big purchase together. Uncle Bob never knew I'd punched his radio to pieces. Until he read this book, of course. Sorry, Uncle Bob!

But that was later in the week. On Wednesday morning, Erin and I were stuck with one station and one song. I can't remember what it was, but it was perfectly awful.

At the Java Room, I lifted myself out of the car with my crutches and walked across the parking lot. The Forefathers Burial Ground (founded 1655) was behind me, but I kept my eye on each step. Up the ramp to the sidewalk. Over the doorjamb. Erin moved chairs out of the way so I could get to a table. It took a while, one step at a time. The place was half full, and I could feel people watching me.

"Can you get me . . . do they have turkey sandwiches?" I asked Erin, once I was in my seat and arranging my crutches.

"Well, it's nine in the morning."

"Could you ask?"

"Do you want coffee?"

"I don't know. Do they have orange juice?"

I had never been out on my legs in public before. Surprising, right? I had walked miles, ten feet at a time, and I had walked ten minutes at a stretch, but that was only at Spaulding or Mom's apartment. I had never subjected myself to my normal life before: the one I had been working toward and dreaming about and dreading for almost five months.

It wasn't so bad.

Erin brought me the turkey sandwich and orange juice. She had a coffee. We sat in the Java Room and talked. I told her how much I appreciated everything she was doing for me. I told her how much I respected her. I told her that she wasn't alone. Yes, I was afraid, just like her, but I was committed.

"I want you in my life," I told her, "not because you are here, but because you are the best and strongest person I have ever known."

We talked about how I could help her. We talked about expectations and responsibilities. We discussed the book. It was stressing everyone out, especially Erin. She wasn't comfortable with the idea of sharing our life.

"Does it have to be now, Jeff? It feels like we're in the middle of this."

That was one thing the agent had told us. If I wanted to write a book, and I wanted people to read it, I had to write it now. *While the memory is fresh*, he said. He meant the world's memory, not mine.

"What if your…PTSD…"

"I don't have PTSD."

"What if things get worse?"

I reached out and took Erin's hand. "Don't worry, my magical wonderful," I said. "Things are going to keep getting better and better."

We talked about the bombing, and what we'd been through. That was the morning I said I wasn't angry at the Tsarnaev brothers. I don't think I'd ever said it before, or even realized it. There was a place inside, maybe, that I was trying to ignore. And when I finally reached down there, and I thought about them…it wasn't anger that came up. It was empathy. We were all in this together, even the bombers, and it sucked for everyone.

"I'd like to talk to him," I told Erin. "Just sit down in his jail cell and hear what he had to say." I tried to imagine it, but I couldn't. I had no idea what that kid would say to me. I didn't know him at all. "I guess that's never going to happen." I laughed. "I doubt his lawyer would think that was a good idea."

We chatted for half an hour or so, until it was time to leave. We had somewhere to be, but I can't remember where.

"I should have had an egg sandwich," I said, as I balanced myself on my crutches. "Who has turkey for breakfast?"

Erin laughed as she cleared chairs to make a path to the door. I worked my way across the restaurant, then out to the sidewalk. When I reached the car, I realized there was a curb. It was at least a six-inch drop. I had walked around to the handicap slope to get in, but it was on the other side of the parking lot now.

Erin hadn't noticed. She was chatting away. But when she saw me looking down, she stopped.

"I can do this," I said.

"Do you want help?"

"No. I can do this."

I put my crutches down at the parking lot level. I leaned forward, working the toes of my right shoe over the edge of the drop, just like Michelle had taught me. I stared over the edge, thinking through the motions. I lifted my left foot and swung it forward. My momentum swung with it, so instinctively I leaned back, and then I was falling backward, my crutches coming out from under me, and I finally learned the true value of the legs. I was out of control, but they cradled me, easing me slowly to the sidewalk. Falling didn't hurt. It felt like I had simply sat down.

"Are you okay?" Erin asked, rushing to my side.

"I'm fine."

She grabbed my arm by instinct, ready to pull me up.

"I'm fine. Just let me rest." I looked around. I was sitting on the curb a few feet from our borrowed Jetta. "I'm going to scoot over to the car," I told her, "and pull myself up."

I worked my way over, grabbed the wheel well, and pulled. I was stronger, but I wasn't that strong. I pulled again.

"Can you give me a hand?" I asked Erin.

Michelle and I laughed about it when I told her the story at physical therapy the next day. "What made you think you could manage a curb?" she said.

"I don't know." I laughed. "I can do a stair or two here, so I thought..."

"But there's a railing here."

"I had my crutches."

"Crutches are different than a railing. Crutches are much harder."

I shrugged. "I got cocky, I guess," I said with a smile. I felt great about the whole thing. Even when it happened, I didn't feel embarrassed. Erin was worried. As she helped lift me onto my crutches, then into the car, she was quiet.

"You okay?" she asked finally.

"I'm great, Erin," I said, fiddling with the broken radio. "It was just one missed step. It didn't hurt me at all."

———————

Three weeks later, we finally closed on our house. We were so excited, we went straight to Costco. As soon as you have that first house, you have to get that thousand-pack of toilet paper, right?

While we were there, Mom and Aunt Jenn called. "It looks like the electricity hasn't been turned on at your house," Mom said.

"Are they . . . !"

I signaled Erin not to worry, that I had it under control. "Mom," I said, "you guys better be gone when we get there. You can come by tomorrow."

When we arrived half an hour later, a basket of mums from Mom and Aunt Jenn was waiting for us on the front porch, along with a bucket for beer from a cousin. It was a beautiful fall day. The leaves were at the height of their color.

I kissed Erin. "We made it," I said.

Then I swung my legs over the edge of the car seat, transferred to the first step outside the front door of my very own house, and hauled myself to the top with my hands. Erin came around with my wheelchair. She unlocked the door. She helped me inside, held the wheelchair as I lifted myself into it, and together, we rolled into our new life.

Big D came by with our furniture a few hours later. We only owned three things: a bed, a dresser, and a chair. So we put the bed in the living room, started a fire in the fireplace, and, as the sun went down and the cold moved in, Erin and I snuggled under the covers and watched *The King's Speech*.

I hadn't made my goal, at least not the one of walking up the stairs into my new life. My sockets were hurting so badly, I could barely put them on. But that didn't mean I wasn't stronger. I was strong as an ox. And I had tried. I had worked harder for six months than I'd ever worked before. In the end, something out of my control went wrong, and I needed Erin's help, but there's nothing wrong with that. No man is an island, right? Who said that, Darrelle Revis?

Ha, ha. Just kidding. It was a poet, right? Erin probably knows. And I'm not afraid to ask her, because admitting your limitations, and accepting help, makes you stronger, too.

SIX MONTHS AFTER THE BOMBING

——◆——

October 30, 2013

Around noon, Erin drove me down to Kevin's row house in the city. I called when we were a few blocks away and told him we were almost there. Five minutes later, he called back.

"Where are you? I don't see Erin's car."

"I'm coming," I said. "Erin dropped me off at the corner."

Seconds later, I heard yelling. Kevin had run out onto his front stoop, and he was cheering for me.

"Shut up, Kevin," I said with a laugh. "I'm trying to concentrate." The sidewalk on Kevin's block was made of bricks. It was uneven, with popped bricks and gaps all over the place. I needed to focus on every step, but Kevin kept cheering, and that brought other people out onto their stoops, and they started shouting at me, too.

"Where's your wheelchair?" Kevin asked, when I stopped at the bottom of his steps.

"I left it at home."

I handed him my crutches, then grabbed his railing and walked up the stairs. I had spent a hundred hours with Kevin in the last six months, but this was the first time I'd made it into his house.

Erin came up a few minutes later, after parking the car, and we took Kevin's convertible BMW to Fenway. It was my first time in his convertible, too, since the trunk was too small for my wheelchair. The Red Sox people were there to greet me, and I walked up the ramp from the players' parking lot to the elevator. I had gotten my new suction sockets the week before. They fit like gloves—like Dan Marino Isotoner Gloves. I had been dragging two loose-fitting doors for a month. As the fit was getting worse, I was falling apart. But all along, I'd been gaining strength. And once the pieces fit, the work paid off. I stood right up and started to walk.

I walked to Kevin's row house. I walked to the elevator. I walked around the stadium from home plate to first base. This was the top level, the one for the press box and suites, so there weren't many fans around, but I shook a few hands. My friends Jess and Pat were waiting in our box. When the Red Sox invited me to the game, that was my condition: I wanted Jess and Pat to come, too.

"Jeff!" Jess said. "I didn't know you were walking."

"Oh, I'm walking."

We hugged. They hugged Erin. "Did you see that?" Pat said, pointing to the field. The grounds crew had mowed a huge circle in the center field grass. Inside, also cut into the grass, were the words: B Strong.

We were sharing the box with the 2004 Red Sox, the team that brought a championship to Fenway for the first time in three generations. The team was throwing out the first pitch, so the only other people in the suite were Jason Varitek's wife and their two kids.

"You should go down on the field with them," she said. "You should throw the first pitch, too."

"Thanks," I said, "but I'm already going down for the seventh-inning stretch." James Taylor was singing "America the Beautiful," and he had asked me to be on the field with him.

They came to get us between the sixth and seventh innings: me, Jess and Pat, Carlos, and three other bombing survivors: Karen, Roseann, and Heather. This time, we took the ramp instead of the elevator. It was a long walk, down four levels and then around to the grounds-keeper's entrance, but I felt strong.

"Go Jeff," people were shouting, as they saw us coming. "Way to go, Carlos!"

People were snapping pictures, but I kept my eyes straight ahead, focused on each step. By the time we reached the field level, I was trucking. We slowed down to avoid a crowd, and someone grabbed me by the elbow.

"Can I get a picture with you, Jeff? I'm so proud of you."

I knew it was a bad idea. There were dozens of people, and if I stopped to talk with them, more would arrive, and I'd be standing on my artificial legs all night. But I could never say no. So I was relieved when security hustled toward me, saying we had to get to the field.

A round of applause burst out, with people yelling and cheering.

"Thank you, Boston," I said. I looked over and saw a group of fans in St. Louis Cardinals jerseys. They were clapping, too.

"Thank you, everyone," I said, nodding toward them. Then I smiled. "Go Sox!"

We had to wait in the groundskeeper's tunnel, a few feet from the field, for a long time. The Sox were leading going into the inning, but the Cardinals loaded the bases, the Sox made a pitching change, and Breslow overthrew third base into center field, giving the Cardinals the lead.

I can say it now, because the Series is over and there's nothing to jinx, but I wasn't worried. The Red Sox had ended the season with the best record in the American League, but nobody thought they were the best team. They lost the first game of the American League Championship series to the Detroit Tigers (probably the best team) and were down by four runs in the eighth inning of the next. Two losses at home, to start a best-of-seven series, would probably have been the end. Then the Sox loaded the bases with two outs, and David "Big Papi" Ortiz hit a screaming line drive to right center field. Torii Hunter, the Detroit Tiger outfielder, leapt to make the catch, barely missed it, and fell headfirst over the wall. Grand slam. Score tied. "Salty" Saltalamacchia got the walk-off hit in the next inning to even the series, and after that, it was all but over.

Sure, the Red Sox were still underdogs. They still had to win six more games, against the best in the world. They were still only ten outs from a crushing defeat, until Big Papi roused them with a fiery dugout speech in the sixth inning of Game 4 in St. Louis.

But the grand slam was the turning point. It was the American minutemen racing down the hill to the Old North Bridge in 1775 and defeating the British in the battle still celebrated on Patriot's Day. You work and work, you get a little better every day, more together, stronger, and then one day something happens, and you believe. Only five people died in Concord in 1775, but a bridge had been crossed, and after that, it was all over except for eight years of brutal war.

Maybe I should end this book with the Red Sox winning the World Series. Big Papi was the MVP, of course, after reaching base 19 times in 25 at bats, one of the greatest individual World Series in history. My boy Salty? He's probably most famous for his throw to third base in Game 3 . . . which skipped into left field and lost the game for the Sox.

Or maybe he's most famous for stopping the victory parade at the finish line of the Boston Marathon, now permanently painted on Boylston Street, and placing the championship trophy there.

I wasn't at the parade. And I wasn't there for Game 6, when the Red Sox won a championship at Fenway for the first time since 1918. The Sox and the Bruins invited me to four games during that summer. The Boston team lost them all. I had to stay home.

But I was there for Game 2 (a Red Sox loss, of course). I was on the field in the middle of the seventh inning, when James Taylor sang "America the Beautiful," and the whole crowd sang along. I didn't have to walk in the marathon next year, I realized then. I was going to walk, no doubt, but it wasn't necessary. I wasn't special. I was only one in the crowd, one of the millions. This was our story, not mine. We were together—the Fenway crowd, Boston, all the good people of the world—and that made us unbreakable.

There was a picture of us, the row of bombing survivors, plus Carlos, in the newspaper the next day. We are lined up along the third-base line, and I'm in the middle, with my crutches in one hand. I'm not even using them for balance. I am just standing there, calmly, like it's nothing.

Like it's no effort at all.

Epilogue: July 23, 2014

I'm working the opening shift at Costco, so I walk out the door about the same time as all the other commuters, coffee in hand. It's a half-hour drive to the store, probably longer in rush-hour traffic, but that's not a problem. I've been doing this for more than a month, and I'm used to driving with my artificial legs.

I'm used to walking on them, too. That doesn't mean I'm happy about it, or that everything is easy. I still wipe out every once and a while, and I can't work on a slick floor, like the one in the Costco deli. I still attend physical therapy twice a week. But I've adjusted to not having legs. I've accepted it. It's a long road to wherever I'm going, but I know that I'm moving now. And I'm heading in the right direction.

Heavy Kevy hooked me up, I must say. Since I couldn't go back to my old job in the deli—besides the slick floor, there was too much walking and carrying heavy trays—he assigned me to the Majors department, right near the entrance to the store. I spend most of my time now talking to customers about televisions and appliances.

It's a little unfair. The associates (that's what we call customers) are checking out the new eighty-inch, and they hear, "Can I help you?" They turn around, expecting an easy brush-off, but it's "Jeff Bauman!" standing there. They start to say "No thank you," and then their eyes drift down to my legs.

Yep, it's him, I can hear them thinking.

"How are you doing, Jeff?" they ask, reaching out to shake my hand.

I don't tell them the truth: that I'm still not comfortable being out in public so much. My co-workers have been amazing; they haven't just welcomed me back, they've carried me on their shoulders. (Not physically, of course, but emotionally.) They are as happy to have me at work again as I am to be back, and that's saying something, because I love having a job, having a routine, being just another guy.

But I still don't quite feel like that—like a normal dude. I still feel separate, like people are watching me out of the corner of their eye. I mean, do they laugh at my jokes because I'm funny (which I am)? Or is it something they're doing *for* me? And when is this feeling going to fade?

"I'm good," I say, whenever anyone asks. "I'm strong."

Both are true. I started with three-hour shifts. Today I'm doing four, most of it standing on my legs. By the end, I'm physically beat. But I'm a little less worn out and sore, I'm almost sure, than I was last week.

After a late lunch with my friends in the deli, I get in my car and head home, beating the rush-hour traffic. It's summer, but the Red Sox game hasn't started. (They're at Toronto tonight.) The Sox are having a down year, last place at the moment, but it doesn't matter like it used to. I've got other things on my mind.

Erin is waiting for me at home.

And Nora. My baby girl.

We found out about the pregnancy a few weeks after I finished the book in December. We kept it secret as long as we could. We didn't want to tell anyone, really, other than friends and family.

But by the first anniversary of the bombing, Erin was showing. And the news media was descending on Boston. We kept out of the spotlight as much as we could. Last summer, my goal was to walk the Marathon. That's what kept me going on some of my hardest days. I wanted to show the world that the bombers hadn't won.

But when the day finally came, I watched the race from a grandstand near the finish line. The pregnancy had been mentioned in *People* magazine. There was an Associated Press article. Brian Williams had induced Erin to (reluctantly) talk about it on national television. We'd done enough.

So instead of something dramatic, Erin and I stood on the sidelines and cheered with my fellow amputee Adrianne Haslet-Davis and my friend Carlos Arredondo. I'm sure I put my arm around him at some point and thanked him once again for saving my life. And I know I put my hand on Erin's beautiful belly as the runners streamed across the finish line. I felt our baby kicking and thought, *The bombers didn't win. They never even came close.*

Now, three months later, I pull into our gravel driveway and park the car beside the house. I almost leap up the three stairs to the back door. Okay, it feels like leaping, but it's actually a careful climb.

I open the door, and there they are: my magical wonderfuls. Erin is beautiful. I haven't seen her smile this much since the bombing, or maybe even before.

Nora is asleep in her arms. She has Erin's chin and my eyes and a shocking amount of dark brown hair.

"We had a good day," Erin says. "It was quiet."

I sit down at the kitchen counter, and Erin slides our baby into my arms.

Nora Gail Bauman. My little girl. I remember something I said in an interview a few months ago, when the reporter asked me how I felt about the future: "I just want to be a good dad," I said.

I had no idea how true that was. Now that I'm holding Nora, what more could I want?

I have my job. I have my family and friends. I have a house to call my own. Erin is going back to school part time in September; she is going to complete the master's program she had to drop out of when the bombers blew our lives apart. With my flexible schedule, I'll be able to care for Nora when she's in class. I'll be able to hold her just like this and say the world's most precious words: *I love you.*

Nora shifts her weight and shakes her head. For a second, she smiles, and I think, *She read my thoughts.* Then she smacks her lips and settles back to sleep. The smell reaches us soon after.

"You won the lottery," Erin says with her quiet laugh. We have an unspoken agreement that whoever is holding the baby when it happens changes the diaper.

"I won the lottery," I agree, as I stand up carefully on my artificial legs, with my baby in my arms, and walk toward the changing table.

Acknowledgments

Thank you to everyone who saved my life at the Boston Marathon, not just my friend Carlos Arredondo, but everyone who touched my life that day. Thank you to everyone who helped; thank you to everyone who ran to help without knowing if they would be hurt or killed. I would not be here without you.

Thank you to everyone who has supported me in my recovery. Thank you to Dr. Kalish and Dr. Crandell, the staffs at BMC and Spaulding, all the businesses (like Blunch and the Colonnade) and people (like Tanya and Isabel) who gave when my family needed it most, and everyone who sent me their love and prayers. Thank you to Matt Gobeille, who sent me the special guitar, and all you kids with lemonade stands.

Thank you to the Red Sox, Bruins, and Pats. Thank you to every celebrity who reached out to victims and their families, especially James Taylor, Kim Taylor, and Ellyn Kusmin, who treated me so well.

Thank you, Boston! My city. Never broken, only stronger.

Thank you to the people who helped make this book happen: Bret "The Hitman" Witter, Anthony "A-Train" Mattero, Peter "No Nickname" McGuigan, and everyone at Foundry Lit + Media, especially Matt Wise and Kirstin Neuhaus.

Thank you to all the fantastic people at Grand Central: Jamie Raab, Sara Weiss, and Deb Withey in editorial; Ann Twomey, who designed the amazing cover; Jimmy Franco; Emi Battaglia; and Carolyn Kurek, Mark Steven Long, and Giraud Lorber, who turned a bunch of pages into a real book.

I have so many family and friends that I can't possibly list everyone.

So to make it simple, let me just say thanks to my three families: the Baumans, the Joyces, and the Hurleys. I love you all. Even you, Forehead.

Thank you to Katlyn Townsend, who stepped in when we needed her and never stepped away; Kevin "Heavy Kevy" Horst, who is unstoppable; John "Nacho Man" Sullivan; Remy Lawler; Michele Mahoney; United Prosthetics; Carlyn Wells and Michelle Kerr; Tim Rohan and Josh Haner; Kevin Sullivan; Elaine Rogers; Pat and Jess; the Corcoran family; and Ryan Donaher, who helps Erin take the trash to the dump and never lets her buy him lunch.

Thank you to the hundreds of people at Costco who treated me like part of their family, even though most of you didn't know me. Thank you especially to James Sinegal, Craig Jelenek, Maya Holt and the whole Nashua crew, Byron Spear, Will Fifield and his wife, Stephanie, Stacy Thrailkill, Judith Logan, and Pennie Clark Ianniciello, who made me believe this book was possible when I wasn't sure.

Thank you to Chief Ed Deveau, the Watertown Police Department, and all the cops, firemen, first responders, EMTs, bomb techs, and FBI agents. You guys are the real heroes.

And finally, to my magical liege, my E: I am thankful for you every minute of every day, even when I'm playing *MLB: The Show*.

This book was written for my fellow survivors and their families and friends, and in honor of Martin Richard, Krystle Campbell, Lingzi Lu, and Sean Collier.